Praise for Vicky Fox

*I've just downloaded **Time to Repair**.... and I love it. I can completely see how it will be a game changer for so many people. It fits entirely with the ethos of what we're trying to achieve at Move. Massive congratulations!*

Lucy Gossage, Oncologist and co-founder of *5K your way*

Vicky has changed my life! Her gentle and adaptive teaching, forging of a community spirit and understanding of the physical and emotional pains we can face has really enabled me to deal with discomfort and bad days better than I ever thought possible. She's armed me with tools to be kinder to myself despite my condition, which I take off the mat into the rest of life, but her classes are very much a grounding anchor to my week, that have especially kept me sane during lockdown and shielding. Having done longer workshops with her too and benefited from so much of her extra advice I can't thank her or recommend her enough. **Amy**

I have attended yoga classes on and off for 30 years and always manage to think my way through the majority of them. Today, however, Vicky suggested we use a mantra or affirmation on our breath in and another for our breath out. This enabled me to stop any negative or unhelpful thoughts and replace them with positive ones. She also encouraged us to hum on an extended exhalation during relaxation at the end of the session. The combination of these two acts meant I felt more relaxed than ever before and will certainly implement into my practice going forward. Thank you. **Helen**

Having practised yoga with many different teachers, I see that Vicky has the rare qualities of exceptional teachers: she is fully present, heart-centred and dedicated to her students. She is a wonderful listener and brings a warm attention to each person she teaches. After her classes, I feel energised, stronger and calmer physically and emotionally. **Tanja**

In addition to enjoying Vicky's live class so much, I have incorporated many of your techniques into my life. I have a whole routine I do even before I get out of bed and a different routine before I go to sleep. Each movement and idea from class is a gift that I can give myself again and again whenever I need and a couple of times when I've really needed the support, I've even taken a recorded class from her website. **Nicole**

I've just found Vicky's videos for yoga for cancer and lymphatic system, I feel such a weight of worry has been lifted… I've done her 30-minute video and feel like my arm is being relieved already! I finished breast cancer treatment 6 months ago (chemo/mastectomy/lymph node clearance/radiotherapy) and I've started feeling a pressure and tightness in my left arm. I'm wearing a compression arm bandage at night but Vicky's exercises have really helped instantly. **Angela**

Once active treatment finished, I was a wreck mentally and physically. I was left with terrifying anxiety and depression. I found re-entering the real world from the cocoon of cancer treatment, terrifying and lonely. Yoga has supported me to make changes for the better, it's enabled me to develop the self-compassion, courage and resilience needed to make changes in my life that my mind and body were crying out for. It has done this in a way that is gentle, supportive, and protective.

As a result of breast cancer surgery, I now have lymphoedema. I can often start a yoga class with a heavy arm blocked with lymphatic fluid. By the end of a class, I can literally feel the flow of the lymphatic fluid draining from my arm! All done without doing a set of prescribed, confusing, stand-alone exercises for lymphatic drainage.

I always feel different after yoga. I have a perspective in thought. I am balanced in mind. There is flow and openness throughout my body. I am unclogged and ready to continue with my day taking this new balance and openness with me. **Katy**

The doctors provide the medical assistance to help me to heal, but that is only a part of the picture, I have taken a holistic approach to healing, my mind, my body, my emotions and spirit. I take an assortment of supplements, have changed my diet and keep active, as well as other integrative approaches such as mistletoe therapy, acupuncture, Chinese medicine and infrared saunas. However, yoga is very firmly placed in the centre of my holistic approach to keeping my mind and body healthy. If for any reason I miss a session, I feel out of balance.

The mantras are incredible, and I will often use my own words during a practice depending on how I feel, mostly 'happy' and 'healed'. **Diane**

Time to Repair

How yoga can restore body and
mind in 5 minutes a day

Vicky Fox

With a Foreword by
Dr Felicity Groom BM, DCH, MRCGP,
PGCME, DipBSLM IBLM

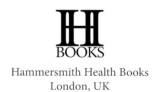

Hammersmith Health Books
London, UK

First published in 2023 by Hammersmith Health Books
– an imprint of Hammersmith Books Limited
4/4A Bloomsbury Square, London WC1A 2RP, UK
www.hammersmithbooks.co.uk

Disclaimer: This book is designed to provide helpful information on the subjects
discussed. It is not meant to be used, nor should it be used, to diagnose or treat any
medical condition. For diagnosis or treatment of any medical problem, consult your own
physician or healthcare provider. The publisher and author are not responsible for any
specific health or allergy needs that may require medical supervision and are not liable
for any damages or negative consequences from any treatment, action, application or
preparation, to any person reading or following the information in this book. References
are provided for informational purposes only and do not constitute endorsement of
any websites or other sources. Readers should be aware that the websites listed in this
book may change. The information and references included are up to date at the time of
writing but given that medical evidence progresses, it may not be up to date at the time
of reading.

British Library Cataloguing in Publication Data: A CIP record of this book is available
from the British Library.

Print ISBN 978-1-78161-240-8
Ebook ISBN 978-1-78161-241-5

Commissioning editor: Georgina Bentliff
Copyediting by: Carolyn White
Typeset by: Julie Bennett of Bespoke Publishing Ltd, UK
Cover design by: Madeline Meckiffe
Cover image by: Merchgraphic/Shutterstock
Heart image (page 29) by: Scarlet Fox
Index: Dr Laurence Errington
Production: Deborah Wehner of Moatvale Press Ltd
Printed and bound by: TJ Books, Cornwall, UK

Contents

Foreword by Dr Felicity Groom   vii
Acknowledgements   ix

1   Taking control 5 minutes at a time   1
2   Union: creating a sense of wholeness to allow your
    body to repair   9
3   Energetics of the body – creating change from within   19
4   Love is everything   29
5   Domes and their role in the health of our body   35
6   Union and the immune system   41
7   The immune system and stress   49
8   Building strength, bones and muscles   55
9   Starting to practise   65
10 Mudras – hand gestures   73
11 Mantras to anchor   79
12 Breathing practices   83
        5-minute savasana   86
        5-minute body scan   87
        5-minute alternate nostril breathing (nadi shodana)   89
        5 minutes to calm (brahmari breathing)   91
        5 minutes to energise (viloma breathing)   92
        5 minutes to cool (sitali breathing)   94
13 Meditation practices   97
        5 minutes' repairing light   97
        5-minute joint space   98
        5-minute heart focus   99
14 Asana practice: supine (with chair options)   101
        5 minutes for digestion   101
        5 minutes for strength   110
        5 minutes to lubricate and flow   120
        If you only have a minute…   129

15	**Asana practice: seated**	**131**
	5 minutes lubricating feet and spine	131
	5 minutes opening face, jaw, neck and shoulders	140
16	**Asana practice: standing**	**149**
	5 minutes' strengthening	149
	5 minutes' hip opening	158
	5 minutes to balance	166
17	**Restorative practices**	**175**
	5 minutes to energise	175
	5 minutes to create maximum space	178
	5 minutes to release tension in the front body	179
	5 minutes to calm and ground	181
18	**Creating a sequence**	**183**
	Begin your day – awakening	183
	End your day – preparing for sleep	189
References		**195**
Glossary of yoga terms		**205**
Index		**211**

Foreword

In her second book, Vicky's extensive knowledge and belief in the power of yoga, along with her desire and zeal to make it accessible to all, are abundantly clear. Amidst our busy and frenetic lifestyles where time is a precious, and sometimes extremely limited commodity, there is growing recognition of the power of lifestyle choices in reversing and preventing a wide variety of chronic diseases. As a GP and a heartfelt Lifestyle Medicine advocate, I am passionate about the importance of healthy habits and their contribution to wellness and longevity. I also feel very strongly that we all should be able to take ownership of our health and wellbeing, working alongside modern medicine and using lifestyle adaptations to help us thrive. As a species, our movement and exercise habits have deteriorated over the years to woefully inadequate levels, made so predominantly by ease of transportation and technological advances. This is despite the overwhelming body of evidence that has consistently and repeatedly shown that exercise provides significant physical and mental health benefits. In addition, people are less able to focus on taking 'time out' to calm and de-stress their lives, contributing to a myriad of health conditions.

As a specialist yoga teacher, Vicky has a detailed knowledge of the body's anatomy and physiological processes, and how these can be impacted by illness. However, she also recognises the time constraints facing many of us and how this often leads to inertia and the inability to initiate change. Vicky leads us through the many health benefits of yoga for our bodies, and beautifully combines easy to understand descriptions with step-by-step instructions for a wide variety of 'bite-size' yoga workouts, bridging the gap between theory and practice, and empowering people to start to incorporate yoga into their lives.

There is no doubt that these 5 minute 'work-outs' will give those that embark upon them the ability to harness Vicky's wealth of expertise and adapt her techniques to their lifestyles. And in doing so, they can be confident that they are gifting themselves with considerable benefits for both their physical and mental health. I have been inspired by her remarkable commitment to her work and am looking forward personally to learning from her teaching. I hope that her readers will enjoy this book as I have, and are able to move forwards equipped with the conviction that significant contributors to health, wellbeing and recovery are well within their control, and that with each small, positive step can come tremendous reward.

Dr Felicity Groom BM, DCH, MRCGP, PGCME, Dɪᴘ BSLM IBLM
GP with a specialist interest in Lifestyle and Integrative Medicine

My gratitude list

My gratitude goes to all my students: without you I would not understand fully the power of yoga. Thank you for trusting me, sharing with me and being my best teachers. Thank you to my husband Neil Fox for patiently taking over 150 photos and editing them especially for this book, Scarlet Fox for designing a heart that blossomed with love and compassion, Martha Fox, for 'yogamats' and Jack Fox for your energy and distraction that taught me to be present.

Thank you to all those who contributed and helped make this book happen: Zephyr Wildman, Lucy Gossage and all the 5K Your Way team, Dr Nina Fuller-Shavel, Dr Ali Courage, Dr Felicity Groom, Dr Anisha Patel, Fearne Cotton, Annie Carpenter, Leslie Howard, Jonathan Sattin, Genny Wilkinson Priest, Lauren Phillips, Doug Keller, Golnaz Maleki, Carolyn White and Georgina Bentliff at Hammersmith Health Books, Twanna Doherty and Emma Fisher at Yogamatters and my wonderful friends and family that make my life complete.

Nicola Price thank you for helping me to breathe and let go and, frankly, for just being you.

Vicky Fox

1

Taking control 5 minutes at a time

Our bodies are incredible, constantly repairing themselves and, although we are largely unaware of it, maintaining our health on a daily basis. Sometimes, however, they need some external help with that process; this might be in the form of surgery, medication or other medical intervention which means for a period of time we become a patient. Patients are often removed from decision-making processes whilst experts decide what to do and how to fix problems. In these periods we can experience a sense of not being in control, of waiting and being in limbo, of being frightened or intimidated, or of feeling confused by language and medical terms that we don't fully understand. Scans and tests can be noisy, stressful and scary (see 'scanxiety' – page 50) and sometimes actually worse than the problem itself. Then there is more waiting for the results of tests, which is all out of our hands and in those of medical professionals and the healthcare services. Things are happening to you, and you might not feel empowered nor sense that you are a co-crafter of your wellbeing. However, although we might need the expertise of medical professionals, the only person who truly knows what it is like to be you, is you. You are unique.

In a period after surgery or treatment when we are recovering, our body might need more assistance or support to go about doing what it does best – trying to bring itself back into balance and repair itself. Even if medical treatment is ongoing, we can assist our body not just by moving and strengthening it, but also by resting and restoring. In this book, we will explore the power of being a human *being* rather than a human *doing*. You, as the CEO of you, can take an active role in helping your body to repair.

The power of yoga to restore us

Integrating yoga into part of your long-term healthcare plan is one way to help you take back some control. Incorporating yoga into your life is a challenge that gives meaning and direction to life but also can give you time to tap into the more instinctive and intuitive layers of your existence, to see your body, mind and spirit as an interconnected whole and repair the whole.

As a yoga teacher specialising in teaching anyone impacted by cancer, I regularly see and hear from students how yoga has helped them recover from surgery or has supported them during their treatment. The empowering benefits of yoga are what I want to share with you so that you can experience something that gives you a break from your mind and find some tools to help you stretch and strengthen your physical body. You don't have to feel good to practise yoga but generally people feel better after.

We live in a chronically exhausted and over-stimulated world and in response to this stress our body suspends all unnecessary functions and activates those more essential for our survival. Our thoughts can trigger feelings of anxiety and sometimes we are not able to turn them off. Being unwell can be all-consuming and we can also experience feelings of helplessness which can make it even harder to cope with life. Yoga is such a helpful discipline because it empowers us to take recovery into our own hands – and because this isn't a 'one-size-fits-all' approach you can find the tools that work for *you* and start to create a toolbox of effective practices to help quieten *your* mind, reduce daily stress, improve *your* energy, rejuvenate *your* body and give it a chance to repair.

Studies show that yoga can help with insomnia[1] and anxiety,[2] increase bone density,[3] increase flexibility and range of motion,[4,5,6] reduce inflammation,[7] increase strength and balance,[8,9] reduce pain[10] and boost immunity.[11] Yoga is not limited to physical movement; it is a practice you can do every day, wherever you are and however you are feeling. It involves breathwork, mudras (hand gestures) and meditation as well as asana (physical poses), so all you really need is a beginner's mind and an open heart to practise yoga. Even the physical part of yoga can be broken down into practices that are supine (lying on your back), seated or standing, or fully supported restorative practices, so you can find something that fits your level of energy on any given day.

Little and often

Regularity is key to optimising the body's potential to repair but, when we are unwell, we use up a lot more energy than when we are well. We also use up a lot of energy when we worry as our mind is often somewhere else wishing that things were different or trying to predict what might happen in the future and how we might cope with this imaginary future. So, we do need to be mindful of how we use the precious time and energy we have to put us in the best place to allow this healing to occur. Little and often can help foster a feeling of taking back control, in bite-sized chunks that fit in with our day. Time is therefore a key element of this book as it is something we often don't feel we have enough of, but if we start with realistic goals of little and often, we can create a habit that, with time, grows into a regular practice. Time to repair our miraculous and magical bodies can start to feel less daunting, more practical and perhaps more realistic.

Finding time every day can feel a little intimidating, especially if you have preconceived ideas about how long a yoga practice should be and therefore feel unable to commit or don't have the energy or time for a daily practice. If the one thing that is holding you back from having a daily yoga practice is time, then starting small might make this change more achievable and realistic. Change can be really hard, but we do have the power to make changes in our own life as long as we have the energy and the desire to want to make that change.

After all, yoga is about becoming more flexible – and not just in a physical sense, but more flexible and adaptable to what life throws at us, starting with time. Life can be crazy, and it can be difficult enough just trying to juggle home, work, kids and pets, never mind finding time for yourself. I often ask people, 'How much time do you realistically have for a yoga practice', because there is no point creating a 60-minute sequence if this is going to be an impossible achievement and just add to the daily stresses instead of reducing them. Five minutes seems like a great starting point, so this book is a collection of 5-minute practices that might be more achievable than a 60-minute practice, (although – spoiler alert – if you did put 12 5-minute practices together you *could* create a 60-minute practice).

These 5 minutes of 'me time' might give you a better opportunity to fit yoga into your day because 5 minutes seems a manageable amount of time even for the busiest person. You can select what you would like to gain from your 5 minutes and, as this might change from day to day, there are a selection of varied 5-minute practices so you can adapt to fit each moment, with whatever that moment brings. There is enough pressure in life and enough things to feel guilty about; we don't need to add to that list a pressure to practise yoga.

Does 5 minutes sound like an achievable amount of time to you? What can you give today? How much time do you have and what would you like to gain from your practice? Some days it might just be to be calmer. Other days you might want more strength and resistance to what life is throwing at you. And on other days you might just want to stretch out and release tension held in your physical body. This book has a simple key to help you quickly see what the focus of each practice is, so that you can select the ones that you need. You can scan and find something to strengthen muscles and bones, stimulate the lymphatic system, calm you, or energise and lubricate your joints. The key is explained in more detail in Chapter 9: Starting to practise.

Just 5 minutes of quality time

Yoga can give you the opportunity to take your scattered mind and focus it on just one thing for 5 minutes; imagine how much energy you have for this moment when you are fully present with it. In those 5 minutes you can try some of the tools in this book to bring your body and mind into focus. See which practices give you a chance to pay attention to whatever is happening in the moment. Some days it might be the physical effort of practising yoga that gets your attention and other days it might be breathing, when you have the opportunity to do just one thing. Doing one thing might also just help with the feeling of fatigue we can experience when we spend our day multi-tasking, not actually achieving what we want to achieve because our mind is so scattered and our energy dissipated, spread out in many directions. We can also be really judgmental of our accomplishments or sometimes our lack of accomplishments, which can close off our hearts and lead to us feeling disconnected.

Time to Repair is not about how much we can do; it is more about quality than quantity – having some time in which we are present and fully and wholeheartedly connected and in the moment, when we aren't judging or criticising but having time just to notice the movement of our breath, the sensations in our body and the thoughts that bubble up. It is about time when we can notice all of these things with kindness and compassion and keep an open heart and a beginner's mind to all that we experience. By having an open mind, you will start to make your brain work in a different way.

'Nerve cells that fire together wire together' (Hebb's law)[12]

Repeating something for 5 minutes a day, every day, may just be enough to kick-start a yoga practice that becomes a natural part of your day and as a result develops into a habit. Our brain adapts and changes when it learns new information; this is known as neuroplasticity. Repetition creates new neural pathways, which make it easier to roll out a yoga mat every day for your 5-minute yoga practice and, because yoga affects areas of the brain involved in motivation,[13] this can help you reinforce a daily practice which will strengthen the neural pathways. It's a bit like a car repeatedly driving down the same muddy track – the more the car drives down the track, the deeper the track becomes, and it gets easier and easier to be in that track. Our brain can work in the same way – the more we repeat things the easier they become, but it also becomes harder to create new tracks.

Changing our tracks and our habitual behaviour patterns can be demanding and feel unfamiliar and it is easy to go back to our old habits because change can feel quite scary and unsettling. But if you have picked up this book then you are probably interested in making some changes and making yoga part of your life, so you might already feel that change is an integral and necessary part of life and that, by reading this book right now, you are taking back some control of *your* life and health. Now you can start to direct yourself down new tracks and begin to repeat new positive habits and 'strengthen the community of neurons to support us in remembering it the next time'.[14]

In *The Presence Process*, Michael Brown says that 'routine becomes what the structure of the word reveals, our route in'.[15] Repetition and routine are key. Repeating 5 minutes of yoga every day gives you that *route in* to explore and experience how yoga can make you feel. Who knows what might happen with your routine? It could start to develop into a regular practice which could grow into a 10- or 15-minute practice *if* you start to feel the positive benefits of feeling good after your daily 5 minutes of yoga. That feel-good feeling might even last for a bit of your day or you might keep it throughout your day, and what you learn on the mat you might start to take out into your life, which is where yoga is really most valuable to you. If you can stay steady and calm in challenging yoga poses, breathwork or meditation, then you can apply that in your life, so that next time someone cuts you up, is rude to you or you feel cross, you can find those tools that you already have and use them. Behaving more consciously allows us to respond rather than reacting to situations, moving from discomfort to balance. The possibilities are there for you to explore when you start small. Take baby steps. One day at a time. One 5-minute practice at a time. Who knows what might grow from this? We know that little acorns grow into large oak trees so what might these 5 minutes grow into?

The 5-minute practices are designed so that you can link them together to create a 10-, 15- or 20-minute routine, or even longer practice, depending on how much time you have. In Chapter 17 I have given suggestions for some different sequences that combine 5-minute practices to help to find a balance in your energetic body as well as your physical body (see page 183) so that you can feel energised to start your day and calm to end your day.

Encouraging your body to repair from inside out

In this book I have deliberately chosen to use the word 'repair' instead of healing. This is because I think the word 'heal' needs more explanation and, over the years, there has been a lot of yoga propaganda together with wild unsubstantiated statements about what yoga can do. Some of this I think was to help promote yoga to the western world by claiming many health benefits for it.

'Healing' can also imply that this is something happening from the outside, something that is done to us rather than creating an environment in which our body is able to work on repairing itself from the inside out. And that brings us back to being a patient where we might feel unable to influence our body's natural ability to try to repair.

The word 'healing' comes from the Old English word *'haelan'*, meaning to make whole, sound and well, and I do believe that yoga has the ability to restore the body and create a sense of wholeness at times when we feel fragmented or out of ease. Andrew Weil says 'it is possible to have an inner sense of wholeness, perfection, balance and peace even if the physical body is not perfect'.[16] This is especially true when you look at the yoga tradition of viewing the body as a multi-layered energetic body full of life force that drives us, as I explain in detail in Chapter x. Restoring wholeness is key to repairing so we will explore further, looking at these layers or **koshas** and the **vayus** or winds of energy that move through all of us. (See the Glossary of yoga terms at the end of the book – page 203 – whenever you are unsure of the meaning of a yoga word or phrase.)

Creating time for *you*

To quote D Servan-Shreiber: 'There are many different ways to tell our body it matters, that it is loved and respected, and to get it to sense its own desire to live. The best way is to let it practice what it was designed for: movement and physical activity. Several studies have demonstrated that the regulation and defence mechanisms that contribute to fighting cancer can be directly stimulated by exercise.'[17]

What would your world look like or feel like if you made the choice to change your perspective and made time for yourself? You, and only you, can invest in a new future by making choices that would increase your purpose in life, allowing you to become fully present with this miracle of life and feel truly alive. What would you like more of in life and what would you like less of? Part of choosing to find this time for you might also mean saying no to things. Saying no is a skill you might have to learn in order to help create new neural pathways. How often do you say yes to something when actually you would like to have said no? You might have said yes because you felt it was a duty, or you felt it was hard to say no, or you didn't feel you had a choice. And if you say yes to something, does it mean saying no to yourself? If this is the case, then you definitely need to learn to say no to some things so that you can take control and create time for you. I find if I actually schedule my 'me-time' into my diary it is a physical reminder that I am making space for myself. I am more likely to stick to it and less likely to fill the space with something else. It also makes it easier for me to say no to committing 'my time' to something else.

The practices in this book help us to become more resilient to and accepting of the unpredictable nature of our lives. We can practise not getting stuck in the past, our story of what has happened to us, but equally not fantasising about the future and what might, or might not, lie ahead. Life will still have its ups and downs which we aren't able to change, but we can become more alive and awake to this very moment that we are in right now. Often you will find that *in the moment* things are actually okay. It is our thoughts about our situation that make it hard, upsetting or difficult. With practice we can become more at ease with the way things are and take what we learn on our mat and the attention we give to these practices out into our everyday lives. Through yoga we can learn contentment – being okay with how things are in the moment. Sometimes we can also find a sense of peace, calm or even stillness that is within all of us, even if we don't always feel it. Creating a practice to find compassion, kindness and maybe a sense of inner stability means that when life does knock us off-centre, we might find we can actually stay steady, create a sense of balance and not get completely bowled over by life's difficulties. I think this also can give us a sense of freedom to be in the moment, not knowing what will come next but just allowing each moment to be.

2

Union: creating a sense of wholeness to allow your body to repair

One

Within us lie the answers
to our deepest questions
and the antidote for all
our fears. The divine
is not an abstraction – it's
as clear and intimate as a
heartbeat or a whisper.

We are penetrated, suffused,
caressed, cell by cell and
synapse by synapse, with
the same love that set
the galaxies to spinning.

No matter how identified
we've become with mind
and body, we can release
the thoughts that blind us
to the truth. Seek the still
point where the words 'you'
and 'I' lose meaning, where
we meet and merge as One.

Danna Faulds from *Go In and In: Poems from the Heart of Yoga*, with permission.[18]

Have you ever wondered 'who am I?'? When you identify with 'you', what is it you identify with? Is it your job, your gender, your body, your qualifications, your race or your socially constructed self? Maybe you identify more with your physical body, or more with your mind? How much of what you know and think about yourself is actually true? How much of what you think is actually based on other people's opinions, views, assumptions and thoughts?

Yoga seeks to unite us and is often translated as 'union' so that we no longer have a sense of 'you' and 'I' as separate but that you and I are actually connected to everything around us. The state of union that is yoga can only be found in the present moment, so pause for a moment, breathe, notice the sounds around you. Notice the smells around you. Observe the feel of your body and the movement of breath in your body. Through our physical sensations we can create a moment-to-moment self-awareness in which we can experience how things actually feel inside of us that is different from our story-telling self-awareness that makes sense of situations based on our personal perspective – depending on our experience of life we may view something in a different way to someone else given we see life through our own lens, which is biased by, and based on, our individual experiences and the assumptions we have made throughout our life.

Evolutionary history tells us that we are supposed to live as part of a tribe, connected to nature and the seasons, using instinct to make decisions and senses like smell to decide if, for example, something is okay to eat instead of reading sell-by dates. As a result of the way we live now we have become separated from our instinctual self, and we can even have a sense of disconnection or fragmentation. The practices in this book can give you a chance to become more aware and to cultivate an inner sense of self or awareness. Awareness is experiencing whatever is occurring in that moment without trying to change, fix, judge, label or interpret it. In Peter Levine's fabulous book on healing trauma, he says that 'people who are more in touch with their natural selves tend to fare better when it comes to trauma' and that 'many seemingly benign situations can be traumatic… hospitalisations and medical procedures routinely produce traumatic results'.[19]

In *The Taittiriya – Upanishad*,[20] an ancient yoga text, a human being is described as having five sheaths or layers, or 'koshas'. These are:

1. a physical layer
2. a breath or energetic layer
3. a mind or mental layer
4. an intuitive layer
5. a bliss layer.

These layers are all linked and affecting one will have a knock-on effect on another layer or layers. Students in my cancer classes often describe a feeling of being hijacked by cancer, that they feel their mind is going in one direction, their body in another, their energy drawn in another direction, and they find it hard to access their intuition as they are often bombarded with too much information. So sometimes these layers of the body are not in alignment, but if we can start to align them, then we can begin to find harmony, bliss and union – not feeling separation from those around us – and with that a sense of compassion and of being fully alive.

According to Candace Pert, neuroscientist and author of *Molecules of Emotion*: 'Most psychologists treat the mind as disembodied, a phenomenon with little or no connection to the physical body. Conversely, physicians treat the body with no regard to the mind or the emotions. But the body and mind are not separate, and we cannot treat one without the other.'[21]

The physical layer of the body

Our physical body is the gross layer that we can palpate and feel and be very attached to and yet also feel disconnected from. When it is said 'you are what you eat' this 'you' refers literally to this physical layer of the body known as the **annamaya kosha**. When we experience illness, injury or surgery, we can either become disconnected from this physical body or find ourselves focusing more on it and identifying with this changing part of ourselves. The physical layer of our body can change dramatically through a cancer diagnosis or through illness and surgery, and how much we identify with it will affect how much we feel a loss of or connection to our identity or sense of self. How much importance you place on your physical body will affect how challenging you find changes to it are.

The energetic layer of the body

'$E = mc^2$: Everything is energy.'[22]

Energy is all around us and within us, vibrating at different frequencies. The physical body was designed to be moved and so not moving it or holding it tightly anywhere can restrict our breathing and the more subtle energy layer of the body, the **pranamaya**

11

kosha. Our physical body is connected from head to feet by connective tissue, the fascia that form a web of connection throughout. Energy or **prana** is distributed throughout the body to our muscles, organs and cells through this connective tissue which holds a complex system of energy channels. Energy is circulated around the body through thousands of pathways (**nadis**), three main channels of energy (**ida**, **pingala** and **sushumna**) and seven energy centres, known as **chakras**.

Our physical body depends on energy for its wellbeing. We are all born with a universal energy – you only have to spend time with a baby to see that – and it is this energy that unites us, when we choose to be fully present and in the moment. Patsy Rodenburg describes presence as 'the energy that comes from you and connects you to the outside world... being present to life is critical not only to your well-being but also to the well-being of everyone around you. It is an act of community'.[23] This is also hugely important because we all thrive better in a community when we are supported by those around us and are able to support back.

When our energy is depleted, our mind and body are affected and sometimes we describe this feeling as being 'burnt out'. We get our energy from food and water, from nature and from people, although some people can be 'drains' and not 'radiators' of energy, so we need to be mindful of who we spend our time and energy with. We also get energy from our breath. When we breathe in, we draw in prana, a vital energy that nourishes us, and if prana gets stuck or restricted in the physical body then the energy can't flow as freely. Scar tissue can act a little bit like a gate in the physical body, preventing the free-flowing movement of fluids but also the nerve pulses that send signals through the connective tissue out to the periphery of the body. The physical practice of yoga can help to release tensions in muscles and fascia. Fascia is a matrix of connective tissue that connects and holds inner organs in place and is woven through muscles, allowing them to work. It contains sensory nerves that gather information and send it back to the brain; this means it is conscious and responsive in that it is always feeding back information to the brain. Consequently, when we feel a stretch in yoga we are actually feeling what is happening in our fascia. Movements in yoga give us the opportunity to unstick the fascia so we can get the prana to start to move into those previously 'stuck' areas.

Where our awareness goes our energy follows. Attention is like a spotlight that moves around and so if you place your attention on something your energy will go there. So, notice if you are placing your attention or energy in the past, by rehashing things that have been and gone, or if you are directing your energy into the future, anticipating or fantasising about a future you can't control. When we are in the past or the future our energy is not in the present moment and it can get scattered, fractured and dissipated, and this can be exhausting. However, we can start to guide our breathing and energy into areas of the body that we have protected or felt scared to move and direct our attention inwards, focusing our mind on our sensations. Our breathing can also physically massage our body from the inside out, bringing energy into those 'stuck' areas.

Also working from the inside-out are **mantras**; these are often chanted to awaken energy by creating internal vibrations through the sound waves that ripple through and stimulate the body. **Mudras**, or hand gestures, are also used to redirect prana or to concentrate it in one location, stopping it dissipating. We will explore the use of mudras and mantras further in this book (see pages 73 and 79).

How changing our breathing can help us connect

Breathing is something that is very much within our control, and it is the quickest way to change how we feel but it also very much reflects how we feel. Even just by starting to watch our breathing it naturally starts to change and by changing the way we breathe we can influence our blood pressure, heart rate, circulation and digestion.[24]

We can use the physical layer of the body to start to control our breathing. Focusing on our exhale is a good way to experience this because we can use muscles such as the tummy muscles (the rectus abdominus) and muscles between our ribs (intercostal muscles) to force or squeeze air out of our lungs as our primary breathing muscle, the diaphragm, relaxes back into the ribcage reducing the space for the lungs. If your think of your exhale as the start of your cycle of breathing, you can focus on your exhale and allow your breathing to start to become a little deeper; if we are consciously aware of our breathing then we can start to create a smooth rhythm to it which, if practised regularly, will positively impact our body's ability to repair.

When our breathing is calm, our mind starts to calm, and our mind is where we hold perceptions, thoughts, assumptions, ideas and conclusions that can keep us stuck. We often live by comparison, comparing ourselves with others as either better or worse, or maybe the same. Often, we judge and label people and things, but if we can connect more deeply, our true nature or true self sees everyone and everything as equal. In this place we are able to realise that joy is possible as happiness is already within us and, although we think that it is things *outside of us* that create happiness, actually they just trigger the happiness that is already there. When we can be aware of

13

our inner experience and befriend what is happening, then we can start to feel more in control and more confident that we are able to change. We learn to be a co-crafter of our wellbeing.

The mind or mental layer of the body

Our mind is where we process all our thoughts and feelings but if we don't digest or process our experiences fully then they can get stuck in the physical body. So, the next layer of the body, the **manomaya kosha**, will be affected by the physical body and the breath or energetic body. Often in yoga we start by stopping. Stopping whatever we were doing before class and creating space to observe and become curious about what is going on in our body, breath and mind. The advantage of noticing at the beginning of the class how we feel on these many levels is that it allows us to observe any changes at the end of our practice and we can see and feel the effects of our yoga practice. We might notice our prevailing mood, levels of energy and what thoughts are going on right now, if our thoughts are pleasant, unpleasant or neutral, and if we are lost in our thoughts and existing on autopilot. We might notice if we are scared or angry, tired or sorrowful. We might notice that when we are scared or anxious our breathing will become more rapid, or we might hold our breath and our physical body will tense, which creates restrictions that we can feel in our physical body. When we make changes in our mind this will influence the physical and energetic body. As awareness is the first step to change, just being aware of our thoughts and the quality of our thinking is the start to becoming more present, in the moment, and less like a sleepwalker moving through our own life.

You may have also experienced a feeling of being 'tired and wired' where your physical body is exhausted, but your mind is busy and active? You go to bed but can't sleep because it is hard to quieten your mind for long enough to fall asleep. Whenever we worry, we are projecting fearfully into an imaginary future and, as we don't know what the future will bring, this is incredibly hard to cope with because it doesn't exist; it is imaginary. It may happen in the future but equally it may never happen. We often think in loop cycles where we recycle lots of thoughts and, if we are in a particular mood, we heighten that thought cycle.

Our busy mind is often what keeps us awake at night and makes it hard for us to fall asleep, but the practice of yoga can give us something else to focus on. Instead of our thoughts we can find other anchors into the present moment. Scanning through our physical body, repeating mantras or watching our breathing are all techniques we can use to centre our buzzing mind. Our body is very much in the here and now even if our mind is careering off elsewhere. We can bring our attention to sensations in the body and guide it away from our thoughts and put them into the present moment of whatever we are noticing in our body. We take our body and our breath everywhere we go, it's free of charge to breathe and so all we need to do is learn some tools that might help us move our attention elsewhere to find some space between our thoughts, and that might just give us a chance to relax and sleep.

Our mind is designed to wander, constantly looking out for dangers so we also try to practise observing our thoughts without judgment. After all, the mind is just doing what the mind does. Therefore, we want to watch our thoughts without pushing them away or trying to block them but just simply notice them, and as we notice we are 'having a thought' we can then come back to watching our breathing, without feeling frustrated. This is a constant process: thoughts bubbling up, noticing them, not labelling them as good or bad, creating more thoughts, but coming back to the breath – breathing in and breathing out. For me, yoga is a process of making my mind quieter for long enough to start to see my innermost nature and what aspects of it are positive and constructive and which are negative and destructive. Then I can work out what I choose to keep and what I want to let go of. This is a 'work in progress' process, a constant practice that is way more challenging than the physical practice of yoga called **asana** (meaning seat). When we connect to what truly is right in this moment, take a breath and find relief from all things that might be and might never be, we realise that this is really the only place that we *can* be in. We suffer when our mind is engaged with what happened in the past and we suffer when it imagines what might happen in the future. So, to reduce our suffering it is truly advantageous to spend as much time as we can in the present moment or just to be aware that we have a choice.

The most fascinating holistic account of how quietening our mind can help us experience a sense of connectedness to everything around us comes from neuroscientist Dr Jill Bolte Taylor's account of experiencing a stroke.[25] Her severe haemorrhage in the left hemisphere of her brain meant she started to lose the ability to speak, write, read and walk. But with the left hemisphere's judgment and chatter quietened she was able to experience herself as a blissful body of energy, connected to the energetic world around her. She writes, 'We are trillions upon trillions of particles in soft vibration. Everything around us, among us, within us and between us is made up of atoms and molecules vibrating in space... I was simply a being of light radiating light into the world. In the absence of my left hemisphere's negative judgment, I perceived myself as perfect, whole and beautiful just the way I was'. How awesome is that?! Her writing and Ted talk were a huge inspiration for me to want to learn more about meditation and make it a daily practice. She had no choice with what happened to her, but I know that I can choose to find some tools that help me become truly present and some space and perspective on things and maybe, just maybe, get that sense of connectedness to everything and everyone around me.

The intuitive layer of the body

In many Buddhist texts the mind is compared to a garden full of weeds and flowers.[26] We have a choice as to what we can plant in our mind – weeds or flowers. What are we going to feed or water in our garden? As we are the gardener, we can also pull out the mental weeds so that our flowers of wisdom can grow. By using our breath to be in this moment and by quietening our mind, we can sometimes hear these 'flowers' speak. There is a saying, which is widely attributed to the 13th century Persian poet Rumi, 'There is a voice that doesn't use words. Listen'. If we can quieten down the judgments, labels and thoughts (mental weeds) we might just get a sense of intuition or wisdom that comes from deep inside and this layer of the body is known as the **vijnyanamaya kosha**. This higher mind has an understanding independent from the brain. Have you ever had a sense of something that logic couldn't explain? This inner intuition is often felt in the physical body. We describe this as having a 'gut feeling about something' or as 'going with our heart and not our head'; we feel 'sick to our stomach' when we hear something awful or upsetting and experience 'butterflies' when we are nervous or stressed; the loss of a person can literally be felt in the heart and we describe this feeling as being 'heart-broken'.

'Listening' to your intuitive body might give some insight into what it is your body needs, in that moment, to help it to repair. In Kelly A Turner's book *Radical Remission*[27], the author describes how she discovered nine key factors that radical remission survivors attributed to their unexpected recovery and that following their intuition was one key common factor. Her research showed that our body innately and intuitively knows how to heal and that trusting our intuition, rather than our analytical brain, often gives us a better insight into what we need to do to help our body repair. Taking time to repair might give you that quiet time to tune in and potentially 'hear' that insightful and intuitive guidance from within, whether you sense it as a gut reaction or a sixth sense that guides you to find answers on what your body needs in order to put it in the best place to nourish and repair. This then naturally leads to two of Kelly Turner's other factors for unexpected remission: one is empowering yourself, becoming the CEO of your body, the driver and not the passenger; the second is deepening your spiritual connection which brings you to the next layer of the body, the **anandamaya kosha** or bliss body.

The bliss layer of the body

'Ananda' means bliss, which might be something you experience at the end of a yoga practice where you can feel a sense of peace, stillness or serenity deep inside. A sense of your true nature, the bit inside of you that doesn't change, is constant, compassionate and connected. You might have a sense of contentment or just of feeling better at the end of your yoga class than you did at the beginning when you first lay/sat on your mat to stop and observe yourself. This may just allow you to feel more comfortable in this forever changing, multi-layered body and to be able to accept changes with a sense of kindness or love.

The interconnectedness of the layers of the body

The koshas view of the body as not just a physical body but one consisting of many connected layers that lead to this bliss body, the deepest layer of yourself, is important because they all affect each other. If moving the physical body affects the breath and energetic flow of the body which calms the mind, this can then allow you to connect to a deep layer of self that is said to be inherently peaceful, calm and connected to all beings. This also works the other way – being connected and calm can have the same knock-on effect on the physical body, energetic body and mental body, allowing it to be in the best place for repairing.

When our physical yoga practice or asana is a mindful practice moving with the breath, staying present, then it becomes a more contemplative practice and integrates these sheaths or layers. We recognise that things might not be the same but that is okay. We are not in control of what life brings us, but we are in control of how we respond, and we might just find through illness or changes in life that we learn more about who we truly are and that how we view life affects how we feel on many layers.

3

Energetics of the body – creating change from within

According to yoga tradition the body is an energy field. The *Hatha Yoga Pradipika*,[28] a 15th century manual on yoga written by Svatmarama, speaks of 72,000 nadis or energy channels that carry energy or prana throughout the body. The main energy channel runs along the spinal column, is known as the **sushumna nadi** and ends at the base of the nose between the two nostrils. There are two other energy channels that swirl and spiral around the main channel. One runs to the end of the left nostril and is known as **ida**; the one that runs to the end of the right nostril is known as **pingala**.

We can also see this energy field when we look at the nervous system constantly relaying information between the central nervous system and the rest of the body. Like the nadis it is extensive and complex, allowing communication of millions of chemical and electrical signals that travel around this intricate nerve network. When we look at our body through this viewpoint, we are literally alive with electricity, pulsing with energy or prana. You may have experienced moments in life when you felt this pulse of life jolting through your body like electricity, like the feeling of falling in love.

The prana vayus

This inner system of energy channels mobilises the body, moving prana into all parts of the body to allow them to function fully. The energy can be divided into five sub-energies known as vayus, often translated as winds. Vayu comes from the root 'va' meaning 'motion' or 'flow'. The five vayus that move in different directions are **prana**, **apana**, **samana**, **vyana** and **udana** and they allow energy to move throughout the whole body. If one of the vayus is not flowing freely or gets blocked, then energy also can get stuck. Our yoga practice can help us free tensions in the physical body and help the subtle movement of energy so that we are at ease as opposed to 'dis-ease'.

Prana vayu

Prana is the wind of energy that we hear about most in yoga. It is a forward and upward-moving energy that is expansive. We get our energy from food and water, people, nature and also from our breath. We can survive without food and water for periods of time, but we cannot survive without breath. This makes it quite a miracle if you stop and think about it for a moment. Prana is connected to the sun which, like our breath, gives us energy and is constantly giving life – without the sun we wouldn't have any life and the same is true of our breath. If an average breath count or respiratory rate is between 12 and 20 per minute,[29] then we have around 23,000 cycles of breath per day. Keeping a normal respiratory rate plays an important part in maintaining the balance of oxygen and carbon dioxide in the body (carbon dioxide is leaving the lungs at the same rate that the body produces it). How we breathe can change how we feel and, by focusing on our inhale, we can use our breath to increase our intake of prana. Prana is active all the time and energises all the koshas or layers in the body (described in the previous chapter). Circulation of the blood in the body and our breathing are all maintained by prana. When we focus our attention on the internal sensations of our body, like our heart beating and the flow of breath in and out, we become very aware of prana, maybe sensing that this is a life-giving force or energy without which we wouldn't have the sensations of being in a living body.

When we worry and experience stress, we use up a lot of energy, fearfully projecting forward into the imaginary future, which can lead us to feeling fatigued and exhausted. Part of the practice of yoga is becoming present with our experiences and not getting hooked by the mind which can lead us to places we don't want to go to or weren't even aware we were going to. By learning some tools to help us with anxiety, or 'scanxiety' (see page 50), we might find we have more energy for being in the moment, for living in the here and now.

Focusing on practices that cultivate more prana might also benefit areas of the upper body such as the chest, lungs and breast. A side effect of chemotherapy and other types of medication is fatigue, so focusing on prana can be beneficial to alleviate symptoms of fatigue. We can also invite more prana into the body not only in our breath but through whole foods, being in nature and being with people who have more prana – those friends who are radiators, whose presence energises us, rather than those that drain us!

Apana vayu

Supporting this upward or forward movement of energy is the downward and outward movement of energy of exhalation and elimination. This energy is apana and is essential for physical downward movements like defaecation, urination and menstruation but also for the elimination of toxins and for letting go of other things we might be holding onto that aren't helpful or serving any purpose. A good example of things that don't really serve us are those thoughts, opinions and views that aren't helpful, that judge and go round and round in a loop in our head using up valuable energy. Can you make a big exhale and let go of any thought right now that isn't supporting you? After all, one of the things we are in control of is our current thought. We can choose to follow the thought or exhale and let it go. Sense also how an exhale can ground us and root us to the earth. Exhaling is a fantastic way of releasing and letting go.

We actually do this naturally without thinking about it by sighing when we are frustrated, worried or even relieved. We sometimes sigh at the end of a long challenging conversation or a hard day at work. Sighing might also be a way to bring our breathing back to a normal pattern when we have been holding our breath, which we sometimes do when we are waiting for something to be over. Or maybe we have been breathing erratically, which can be a response to any stress or anxiety we are experiencing?

When we do lengthen our exhale, this stimulates the parasympathetic side of the nervous system. You can feel this for yourself by taking your pulse whilst you breathe in and out. When we breathe in, our pulse rate speeds up and when we breathe out our pulse rate slows down; this slowing down is also known as 'rest and digest'. It is called this as when we dial more into the parasympathetic side of the nervous system the body goes back to digesting fully. Other systems, like the immune system, also benefit and start to function fully in 'rest and digest', and as apana focuses on elimination and detoxification it also supports the immune system and the body's ability to defend itself against outside invaders like bacteria or viruses and remove them from our body.

Practices that focus on apana could benefit anything in the reproductive system (ovaries, uterus, prostate), urinary system (bladder) and colorectal system. They could also be beneficial for any side effects of constipation, nausea or fatigue.

Samana vayu

When we breathe in, we are powered by the energy of the sun and prana, and when we breathe out, we are grounded and connected to the earth and apana. When you breathe in and breathe out you might start to be aware of the pauses in between the breaths. When you breathe in you might sense or notice a pause at the top of the inhalation before you breathe out. When you breathe out there is a pause at the end of the exhalation before you breathe in. Here in the pause is the spacious and equalising energy of **samana** and we can work with breathing in and out to an equal ratio to stimulate radiating, pulsing samana that draws energy to the centre of the body.

Prana and **pranayama**[30] describe this energy as more of a swinging pendulum moving from side to side. 'Saman' means 'balanced' and this energy supports healthy digestion of food but also experiences and memories. When working fully, samana helps us to fully digest life experiences without leaving behind any toxic residue. It works in conjunction with our digestive fire known as **jatharagni**. Jatharagni brings us energy and life as we digest our food and is the divine fire that is in all of us. This energy motivates us and can give us a confidence or a power that comes from deep within which we refer to as 'gut strength' or someone with that strength as 'having guts'. Samana helps to balance the energies of prana and apana, and, like apana when we start to calm the nervous system, we can help the body move back towards resting and digesting and away from fighting or fleeing.

Practices that focus on samana can benefit areas of the body such as the stomach, liver, pancreas, kidneys and gallbladder. We will explore the digestive system more in Chapter 6 on the immune system, and many of the 5-minute sequences in the book focus on digestive health and stimulating samana energy.

Vyana vayu

Vyana is an expansive energy that distributes energy out to the periphery of the body – the arms, legs, fingers and toes. Expanding out from the heart, this all-pervading vital energy of the heart and lungs governs circulation. It moves outwards along the many nadis. According to Rol Sovik in *Moving Inwards: the Journey to Meditation*,[31] vyana 'induces the movement of blood, lymph and nervous impulses'. When we are exhausted but experience a second wind of energy this is also vyana.

Practices focusing on dispersing energy out into the limbs and the circulation could be beneficial for any side effects that affect the muscles, limbs, nervous system, blood and bones. You will find yoga sequences for lymph flow and lubrication that focus on releasing scar tissue and tight connective tissue so that the joints in the body can move more freely and as a result so can blood, lymph and nerve impulses. When we move our body in yoga, or when we visualise moving our body or moving breath and energy through our body (see Chapter 13: Meditation practices) we help to stimulate vyana vayu and unite the whole of our body with energy.

Udana vayu

Udana helps prana with inhalation and exhalation and the functions of throat and mouth, which also allows energy to flow from the heart to the head. Our ability to speak our mind, to express ourselves and be fully authentic in the way we speak comes from the energy of udana. Being able to speak up and communicate and find our own voice is important when recovering from illness and repairing. Our gut or intuition might guide us to take control of nourishing ourselves and this might be different to what is expected of us by those around us. Speaking out, taking control can be empowering. Said to flow in a circular motion, udana can be viewed as 'spiralling rings of energy'[32] and if it gets blocked it can affect cognition and communication. Stimulating udana can be beneficial for thyroid, larynx, eyes, brain and throat.

We will explore further the use of sound in mantras and how the vibrations that the sound creates can ripple out into the body, massaging the internal organs from the inside of the body out. You can feel this yourself if you take your hand gently to your throat and make a 'mmm' sound as you exhale – you will feel the gentle vibration that the sound makes. This simple way to stimulate udana vayu can be used with any of the 5-minute practices and, because humming naturally lengthens our exhale, it also helps to calm the nervous system, which allows us to 'rest, digest and repair'. You can explore making different sounds to see if one particular sound helps to free your throat and your voice and allows you to fully express yourself. What does it feel like to have an all-powerful voice and to be authentic and honest in how you express yourself?

Stimulating the vayus

A lot of the yoga postures stimulate all the vayus but some sequences will focus more on one so that you can tailor the practice to focus on one of the movements of energy. In Chapter 10 on mudras (hand gestures) you can find specific mudras that are said to focus on certain movements or winds of energy so you can add a mudra into your practice or into your day and explore in your own multi-layered body what the benefits are to you of a particular hand gesture.

Some days we can just feel generally low on energy and not like doing anything. The best thing we can do for fatigue is to move our body, and some of the practices in this book focus more on energising, so look out for the Ⓔ that shows the practices that help to energise.

Energetic centres

The subtle energy of the body is also seen as moving through different energy centres, or wheels known as **chakras**. Chakras are said to pull energy in from around us and distribute it through the body. If the energy does not move through these chakras then it can get stuck and, if one is out of balance, then the whole energetic system is out of balance. Again, this might be described as 'dis-ease' as opposed to the system working 'at-ease'. Each energetic centre is said to have its own vibration and ideally, we are trying to get all of the chakras to be in balance with each other.

Muladhara chakra

The first of the chakras, known as the root or **muladhara** chakra, is said to be where the vital energy of the body and spirit dwells like a coiled serpent at the base of the spine. The process of awakening or uncoiling this energy is known as **kundalini**. The term kundalini has become synonymous with a style of yoga but it really refers to awakening this dormant energy at the base of the spine and drawing it up to the crown of the head, balancing the energetic body.

On a physical level, the first chakra relates to feeling rooted or grounded in the feet, legs, bones and base of the spine and is associated with our tribal nature. When this chakra is in balance you feel strong and confident, able to stand up for yourself, and balanced and stable, so that you can stand on your own two feet. Practices to open up the feet and hips help to bring some focus to this lower chakra as do chair poses and warrior poses, which you will find in the 5-minute practices.

The sound associated with this chakra is the sound 'lam' (pronounced 'lum') a bija, or one-syllable seed mantra that has no translation but has its own energy or energetic vibration. You can try chanting this sound and feeling where you sense it resonating and directing the vibrations down into the base of your spine.

Svadisthana chakra

The second chakra, known as **svadisthana**, relates on a physical level to the sexual organs, womb, ovaries, pelvis, bladder and small and large intestines. Located in the sacrum, it also represents fluidity and being able to go with the flow. This is important when trying to create change in your life, so that you can be receptive and open to change, not trying to swim against it but just going with it.

The root sound for this chakra is 'vam' (pronounced 'vum') and you can try chanting this to see where you feel the vibrations of that mantra and if you can sense the sound rippling out to your sacrum like a wave rippling out on water. Hip openers are ways of physically releasing this lower area of the body.

Manipura chakra

In the area between the navel and the rib cage the third chakra relates to the abdomen, stomach, kidneys, adrenal glands, liver, gallbladder and upper intestines and is known as the **manipura** chakra. The diaphragm is in the area of this power chakra that holds these diverse and powerful organs that all have their own energetic qualities. Your kidneys filter out toxins, your liver protects you from harmful substances, your diaphragm helps to expel stale air and toxins and your adrenals are ready to provide you with energy to help you fight or flee. This navel centre of the body, as with samana energy, is also linked to the digestion and the ability to digest fully our experiences in life. When this chakra is open we feel fired up and alive. Practices that work at twisting the body and stimulating the navel centre can release tension held in this area of the physical body.

The one syllable mantra for the third chakra is 'ram', pronounced 'rum'. You can try chanting 'ram' and letting the sounds vibrate down into your belly.

Anahata chakra

The fourth chakra **anahata** is also known as the heart chakra, which we will explore further in Chapter 4. Our heart is a place of compassion, love, vulnerability and strength but also of sorrow and heartache. The ancient yogis saw it as the seat of our soul, and that our soul or **jiva** resides in a cave in our hearts. Learning compassion towards ourselves is key to feeling greater connection, but one of our greatest challenges is often being loving and kind to ourselves. There is great wisdom in the heart and when we are authentic and loving, life just feels like it flows easily. However, some of us mostly identify with the physical external body, the part of us we can see when we look in the mirror. When we believe we are only the body we can see, we work hard to stop that external body from changing and it can be hard to feel contented with it as it changes. But it will continue to change if we are lucky enough to age. My grandma, in her nineties, told me she would look at her reflection and wonder who the old lady was looking back at her because she didn't feel like that old lady inside of herself; inside her heart she still felt young. If we are able to focus more on our heart then we can find that we can connect with others through our hearts and discover a deeper contentment in our hearts and souls, a part of our body that doesn't change, and fully experience living.

Anahata chakra on a physical level relates to the heart and circulatory system, lungs, ribs, breasts, shoulders and arms. When we practise poses that open up the heart, from a physical perspective these would be chest-opening poses where we sense a stretch across the chest or feel our shoulder blades coming closer to each other. However, we can also connect on an energetic level anytime we pause, drop our awareness down to our heart centre, breathe into this area as if we could breathe directly into our chest, and give thanks. Just try asking yourself, 'What am I grateful for today?' and see what pops out of your heart. What is it your heart connects to? We can nourish our hearts by focusing on being kind and compassionate to ourselves. Even by carving out your five minutes for yourself you are practising compassion. Chapter 13 has a heart-based meditation you can try to bring more awareness to this energetic centre (see page 99).

'Yam' (pronounced 'yum') is the mantra of the heart centre. Placing your hands on your heart, chant 'yam' and sense or feel the vibrations at the heart centre. Visualise them rippling out from your heart to others that you love.

Vishuddha chakra

The fifth chakra, the throat chakra known as **vishuddha**, is an energetic centre of expression; it is our communication centre. Our ability to express ourselves fully and be more authentic in the way we speak might mean we become more responsible for our health and take a more active and less compliant role in our wellbeing. It could involve questioning choices and decisions made by others and researching possible alternative treatments, knowing that we have choices and being able to express what those are and standing up for what we believe to be best for us. In this way we can move from being a patient to being in charge of our own destiny. It may be easier to spot when we are not being authentic or able to express what we truly feel? In this moment you may be able to sense this disconnect between what you feel and what you are actually saying. Being aware that this energetic centre might be out of balance or out of ease is the first step to finding that balance. What might be preventing you communicating fully?

Often, we look as though we are listening but actually we are just waiting for our turn to speak, and our mind is focused on our response to what is being said. Listening is not the same as waiting to speak. So take a moment to actually 'hear' what is being said without thinking of your answer. Listening is being present without judgment or preconceived ideas so that you can hear what is actually being said and fully 'see' the person who is speaking to you. Being more authentic in the way that you speak to people might also mean 'speaking up' – being able to ask for help when you need it. If you are recovering from surgery or from an illness your recovery might be aided by the support of friends and family around you. Feel comfortable being honest in telling people how they can help you, tuning in to the next chakra (ajna – see below) to feel intuitively what you need support or help with. Kind people love to be asked to help. It makes them feel useful and we feel good about ourselves when we can support and help others. Make a list of jobs that you need help with, such as support with cooking, picking up kids, driving you somewhere if you can't drive, or posting letters.

Physically the fifth chakra refers also to the mouth, thyroid, teeth and gums and so chanting and singing are wonderful ways to stimulate this chakra. 'Ham' (pronounced 'hum') is the mantra or sound associated with the throat. Try placing a hand on your throat and your other hand on top of that and chant 'ham'. Emphasise the 'mmm' sound in the 'ham' and feel this vibration in the throat while imagining the internal massage of the sound waves at this energetic centre.

Ajna chakra

The energetic centre associated with clarity, intuition and the power of our mind is the sixth chakra, **ajna**. Often called the 'third eye', this is the meeting point of the two energetic streams ida and pingala nadis, where masculine and feminine energies meet and a point where the mind meets the body. Physically it relates to the pineal and pituitary glands, brain, ears, eyes and nervous system. When we are repairing this can be seen as the ability to fully see and hear what is going on inside of ourselves. It might be the ability to tap into our intuition or our sixth sense and trust in our insight and inner wisdom through which we naturally know what is going to help us to repair, nourish and nurture ourselves. We might need to quieten down our constantly chattering mind so that we can hear this inner whisper of wisdom.

We can focus on this point of intuition when we chant 'om', or when we practise **nadi shodana** or alternate nostril breathing or any practices which focus on the third eye.

Sahasrara chakra

The seventh chakra, **sahasrara,** is said to hover above the head. Connecting to this chakra gives us a sense of connection or oneness, that we are spiritual beings navigating a human existence. We have everything we need within us and we don't need to look outwards to experience this, but inside to find true happiness and contentment.

Achieving balance

These chakras all have different vibrations and distinct properties, but yoga reminds us that we are whole, interlinked and connected and that to create a sense of wholeness we need to bring all the energetic centres into balance – to find balance within because if one centre is out of balance then so are all the centres.

4

Love is everything

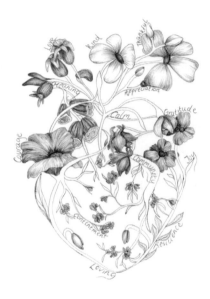

The opening of the heart has a huge role in yoga and lots of yoga practices focus on the heart and cultivating a greater connection with our true nature and thereby a deeper sense of belonging. When we refer to the heart, often it is not the actual anatomical placement of the heart but rather the energetic centre of the heart. However, connecting to our anatomical heart is a great way to be present because the heart is beating in this present moment. When we do connect with our body on a physical level, we might be aware of the thudding of our heart beating inside our chest. Our brain is capable of filtering out the cardiac sensation so that it doesn't interfere with our ability to perceive external sensations, so it is not always easy to be aware of our heart beating, but we definitely have a better chance of noticing these internal sensations when we stop being a 'human doing' and start to be a human being.

By quietening your mind, through breathing and meditation, you are able to turn your senses and awareness inwards (known as **pratyahara**) and you can start to feel what is actually going on *in* your body in that moment and how this may change from moment to moment. The advantage of drawing your awareness inwards is that you observe and feel without reacting. You can reflect on your sensations, which means that you have a pause before you react to them, and it is this pause that allows you to respond to things instead of reacting. We are always better with some space and pauses in life; we are less likely to have a kneejerk reaction to things when we give ourselves space to observe our feelings and sensations in a non-judgmental way. You may have experienced this yourself if you have ever been angry and have responded to a situation by writing a letter or an email. If you re-read that same message later when you have had time to reflect you may realise that you no longer feel quite so strongly as you did when you wrote it. With space and time your response is different.

Quiet centredness can prove very challenging to achieve and you might face resistance, feel stuck or even fearful. This may be the first time you have given yourself time to tune in to what is happening inside of you. You may have deliberately kept busy so that you could keep yourself distracted from what is going on inside of you. Being ill can often be the opportunity to stop the treadmill, so to speak, and start to live life more fully, being more present with the experiences of life, which can be good and bad, joyful and painful and sometimes mundane, repetitive and ordinary. Whatever the experiences are, they are *your* experiences and *your* life. You are the only one who has the power to make changes in your life and this can begin by stopping and feeling fully who you are right now and what it feels like to be in your body today. What sensations are you aware of? Can you sense your heart beating – that steady beating of life inside your body? Can you feel the pulse of blood and fluids in your body? Or maybe just under your skin you can sense the subtle movement of energy in your body?

We looked at vyana vayu (page 36) and udana vayu (page 23) as energies from the heart, and anahata (the fourth chakra – page 25) as the centre or wheel that the energy flows through. Every single one of us has an innate wisdom, strength and power that comes from our heart centre. I see this in the students that I teach and in the way that they overcome and adapt to the challenges in their lives. I see the pain and grief that they feel as a physical sensation of their hearts being broken but I also see how they open up their hearts to being more compassionate to themselves to try to understand how they might be able to support themselves. I see how some live with constant treatment for cancer and the huge courage that they have on a day-to-day basis. It is through your heart centre that you can truly feel what it is to be alive and to live fully.

Love is something that many songs have written about; top-10 hits tell us that 'Love is all around us, it's everywhere we go'[33] and 'All we need is love, love, love. Love is all we need'.[34] We all want to love and be loved, and this is the heart of the human experience. I think we are most content when we are loving and are loved in return. Being loving and kind is our deepest and truest nature but sometimes, when we lose our connection to that true nature, we can behave in a way that isn't loving and kind. We can behave in certain ways out of fear, anger or resentment, but if we can connect to that true sense of self, we can experience our true nature that is loving and kind and from this place we can establish new neural pathways or patterns of behaviour which involve us being kind to ourselves through the nurturing practices of yoga.

When we judge ourselves or others, we actually close our hearts because we can't be open to others and be judging at the same time. So, to be fully loving we need to try to come with a beginner's mind, a sense of neutrality and an open heart.

Fighting talk

Often when we are ill we speak in terms of fighting: we try to 'fight off' infection, we 'battle' diseases, we 'fight back' against an illness, and 'struggle' with a condition; we can even try to 'stamp out' a disease. There are studies looking into 'tackling' type 2 diabetes or 'killing' zombie cells (cells that aren't functioning properly). The metaphors can be useful when fundraising because they ask people to help 'win the war' against a certain disease or chronic condition and this can definitely create a sense of community. We are invited to come together and collectively fight an 'enemy' by contributing financially to the battle. However, for some of us these metaphors can be destructive because if we 'lose the fight', does this imply that maybe we didn't fight hard enough or could have done more? The 'fighting' analogy turns people into winners and losers. Having had more than my fair share of friends and students die from cancer (my special area of expertise), I know that this is most certainly not the case. I have met the bravest and most courageous people impacted by cancer who opened their minds to all possible healing potentialities and did everything they could to help their body heal, but nevertheless they died. Cancer, like most diseases, is complex and the product of many different influences and sometimes there appears to be no rhyme or reason why some people die and some survive, and no amount of 'fighting' could have changed that.

Fighting talk can also stimulate a fight-or-flight response (see page 49) which is not helpful when trying to repair our body. We want our immune system functioning fully and this is not the case when we are in 'fight' mode. Furthermore, do we really need more fear and anger in our world? Or would it actually be more beneficial to add more kindness and love? On that basis, I think any compassion-based practices are hugely beneficial because they take us out of fighting and into loving. The more compassion we can have for ourselves, the more compassion there will be for someone else, who then might be kinder and more compassionate to someone else who is then kind and compassionate to another person... You can see how this can have a knock-on effect. Imagine if everyone was kind. That would be a wonderful world to live in.

Connection

I have spoken about gratitude before in *Yoga for Cancer*.[35] When we have moments of gratitude, we also get moments of connection. We feel less like an island and more like a community when we find people and things we feel grateful for. When things are challenging in life, we may just have to give thanks even if, in that moment, we are not sure what we feel grateful for – just giving thanks and taking a moment to bring our awareness to our beating heart. Then, in the awesome presence of our own life force, we can sense that pulse of life. We all have a heart that beats and everyone we interact with has a heart that beats so we are united by this commonality of a beating heart.

Maybe you feel the pulse of life in your breath, because for as long as we are living, we will all be breathing in and breathing out? We all have this in common – we are living beings breathing in, breathing out.

If feeling gratitude for the miracles inside your body is too demanding, then maybe it's something outside of your body that you could feel thankful for – maybe something in nature? Sometimes you just have to start small, with a bud swelling or a flower blooming. See the colours, and the shape of the petals and how remarkable these are.

Maybe you can picture a tree, with roots that stretch down into the earth and branches that proudly reach out into the sky? Expand outwards to sense the extraordinary beauty of a whole forest of trees. Each tree unique and individual but, like us, they are connected by their roots, hidden beneath the soil. If we choose to, we can see how different we are from each other, but notice how this creates a sense of separation. We can also choose to see how we are the same. We also have these roots that can connect us to each other. We have a choice in how we feel. When we feel different from each other we can feel divided, separate and alone, but when we choose to see our sameness, our oneness, we can also experience the peace and serenity that come with that.

From my experience when I am connected to someone or something, I feel an openness in my heart, I feel less scared and I can relate to what I have in common with others and feel at one. This is quite peaceful and generally makes me feel happier or more contented with my life. I also think we can get that same connection with ourselves when we are able to accept who we are, and this comes again from taking the time to tune into what it feels like to be you in this moment right now – not analysing or judging, criticising or trying to solve anything but just breathing in and breathing out; just being, and not doing.

You can follow the heart-focused meditation in Chapter 13 (page 99) anytime you want to connect to your heart.

5

Domes and their role in the health of our body

In this chapter we will explore how the many domes in our body affect the whole body and therefore the flow of energy, the vayus and the chakras, and, by allowing a relaxed, full movement of these physical muscles, how we can start to stimulate the movement of energy in the subtle body – the body within our physical body. The more we understand our body, the less confusing it will be and the more in control we can feel. We are able to free up tension held in these muscles and allow them to move fully and freely. When these muscles move through their full range of motion, which they can't do if they are held tight or they are weak, then we can have an internal massage of our organs and ducts. If we can enable the body to relax then energy can flow freely, which it can't do if the body is held tight, stuck or rigid. Breathing is the key to letting go, to releasing and to feeling that the body is moving holistically rather than separately.

The respiratory diaphragm

The respiratory diaphragm is a dome-shaped muscle running around the inside of the ribcage. It sits at the bottom of the thoracic cavity and separates your heart and lungs from your abdominal cavity. The respiratory diaphragm can move automatically but it can also be forced or controlled. When we breathe in (prana), the central tendon of the dome pulls down, the belly and the lower ribs expand and air is drawn into the lungs. As the diaphragm moves downwards, it presses down on the abdominal cavity which has nowhere to go but outwards, hence we see, or should see, the belly move when we breathe fully and diaphragmatically.

When we breathe out, the diaphragm moves back up into the ribcage and air is expelled out of the body. This movement also massages the internal organs, because they change shape as the diaphragm presses down on them and increases new blood flow to these areas; this in turn helps with the process of elimination and digestion (apana vayu and samana vayu). The diaphragm helps blood and lymphatic fluid flow from the periphery of the body, such the legs, back up towards the heart against the pull of gravity (vyana vayu).

Our diaphragm can be limited in its movement when we are not breathing fully, or it can also be restricted by poor posture. When we sit slumped with our spine rounded or chest closed (a common position when we are working at a computer or sit for long periods of time relaxed in a chair) this prevents full movement of the diaphragm. Conseqently, not only are we not getting breath in and out of the body, oxygen in and carbon dioxide out, but we are limiting the movement and the awesome massaging quality of our breathing.

I have been really influenced over the last few years by a beautiful soul called Nicola Price who trained me to be an 'inspirational breathworker'. She has introduced me to the importance of letting go through the diaphragm using a conscious, connected breathing technique to remove unhelpful patterns of behaviour and to release deeply held layers of trauma and pain. See the references for details of her website where you can learn more about her work.[36]

Other domes in the body

The respiratory diaphragm should not be seen as a segment but as part of a body system,[37] because, as it moves, other domes in the body respond to that movement (see Figure 1). We have:

- a cranial diaphragm that is composed of differentiated connective tissues in the skull. It helps to maintain pressure in the cranium and controls the flow of cerebrospinal fluid – the fluid that bathes the brain and runs through the spinal column.
- a cervical diaphragm, composed of the tongue, muscles of the hyoid bone and scalene muscles, that controls the pressure between the cervical (neck) spine and cranium. This diaphragm also promotes swallowing and phonation, production of vocal sound and speech (udana vayu). When we breathe in, muscles in the throat lift and open the soft palate, allowing the vocal diaphragm to lift to make space for breath to come in. Sounds or mantras that have an 'aaaah' sound help

to soften the palate and larynx. Conversely, you can observe how making a high 'eeeee' sound creates the opposite feeling of tension around the throat and can also pull the head down and forward, a head position we want to avoid.

- a dome, or diaphragm, at the pelvic floor that supports the bladder, bowels and reproductive organs. This broadens and flattens as you breathe in and domes and rises as you breathe out.

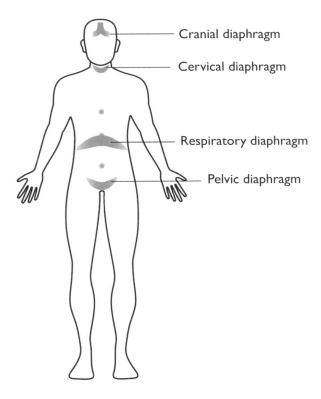

Figure 1 Domes in the body

We know that these domes are linked by connective tissue and, as we breathe in and out, all should respond and move. Leslie Howard puts it beautifully in *Pelvic Liberation*,[38] saying that 'the respiratory and the pelvic systems are intimately connected. Ideally their movements are synced with each other. Considering that we breathe between 17,000 and 20,000 times a day our pelvic health depends on good breathing'.

Our deepest layer of tummy muscle is the transverse abdominal muscle. When we exhale, it starts contracting, increasing the pressure in the abdomen, assisting with our breath out. A healthy pelvic floor moves with this contraction and helps with exhalation.

It is interesting that a continuous sheath of connective tissue links the transverse abdominal muscle and the fibrous sac that surrounds the heart, known as the pericardium (imagine it as being like the peel of an orange). Therefore, when we are breathing fully, using our diaphragm, transverse abdominals and pelvic floor, the movement will have a massaging effect on the heart too.

Strengthening the diaphragm

This is an easy way to connect to your respiratory diaphragm and to encourage movement in all domes:

- Lie on your back with your knees bent, find the neutral spine position (see Figure 5c, page 63) and place a yoga block on your belly above your navel.
- Breathe down into the block and feel the block rise on inhale and fall on exhale.
- Continue breathing down into the block so that you get feedback from the movement of the block. You can also experiment with a small bag of rice on your belly, which creates a bit more resistance to your breathing, and continue breathing into the bag of rice and feeling it rise on inhale and descend on exhale (see Figure 2).
- Try moving the block/bag of rice down to below your navel to explore the movement of breath here. Can you feel the movement of breath into the block/ bag of rice?

If you feel that you are doing the opposite and that your belly draws in on inhale and out on exhale, you are experiencing reverse breathing. This may be as a result of trauma. When we reverse breathe, we aren't breathing in or breathing out fully and often this can create tension in our shoulders, neck and jaw.

If you feel comfortable lying on your tummy, then you can try breathing practices lying face down. Try placing a folded blanket under your forehead and, if lying prone like this is uncomfortable on your lower back, maybe add a folded blanket under your belly (see Figure 3).

Once you are prone you can start to breathe consciously and feel your breath moving into your belly and your belly moving into the blanket or the floor. Awareness is the first step to change, so being aware that you are reverse breathing will be the start of you being able to change your breathing to full diaphragmatic breathing.

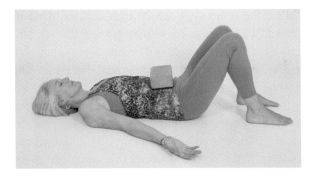

Figure 2 Diaphragmatic breathing with block

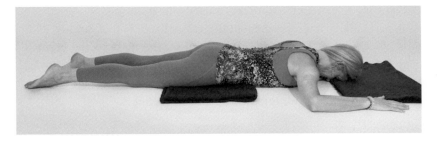

Figure 3 Diaphragmatic breathing prone

The vagus nerve

The vagus nerve is one of 12 cranial nerves – the nerves that connect the head, neck and throat to the brain directly, not via the spinal cord. It regulates heart rhythm and governs the response of the parasympathetic nervous system. (As explained more fully in Chapter 7, the autonomic nervous system that controls the body functions that we do not consciously manage, is divided into the sympathetic and parasympathetic nervous systems. The former puts us on the alert and is responsible for what is known as the 'fight-or-flight' response; the parasympathetic nervous system is associated with rest, recuperation and recovery – what is called 'rest-and-digest' mode.)

The vagus nerve 'wanders' from the brainstem (the stalk at the base of the brain that connects brain to spinal cord) through the chest and the respiratory diaphragm into the abdomen to the digestive system, intestines and organs of elimination. It communicates back to the brain stem which then adjusts to what the vagus nerve perceives about the body. The vagus nerve may sense a threat even if a real threat is not present – for example, when we hold our breath or are not breathing properly, not properly using our diaphragm. Then a message is sent that we are under stress, and we need to prepare our body to respond – we go into fight-or flight mode.

The vagus nerve also runs through the laryngeal muscles in the throat, and picks up on changes in pressure in the respiratory tract. As it runs downwards, passing through the diaphragm, it can be stimulated by breathing fully and diaphragmatically as this increases the pressure on it, telling it that we are in a safe place. When we consciously breathe, as we do in yoga, we are in control of our breathing and, by exhaling, we increase the firing from the vagus nerve to the heart and this decreases our heart rate. Our body dials more into rest-and-digest mode and our body can start repairing and healing, digesting to extract the nutrients it needs for restoring.

What is particularly interesting about the vagus nerve is that 80% of its fibres are 'afferent' – that is, they send messages *back* from the body to the brain – so it is constantly feeding back how we are feeling. Consequently, it helps us to be able to tune in to what it feels like to be us and truly be aware of how we are actually feeling in the moment and not how we think we should be feeling.

6

Union and the immune system

What we call the 'immune system' is really a concept – it is a combination of lots of systems, organs, cells and chemicals that work together to fight infection. This interplay of systems is at work at all times to protect us externally and internally. Our skin is exposed on a daily basis to the external environment, the invisible radiation from the sun, chemicals, bacteria, viruses and other pathogens. It is a flexible, waterproof insulating barrier to the outside world and is packed with immune cells.[39] When you move your body in yoga you stretch your skin and stimulate your circulation, which helps the immune cells to do their job more efficiently.

The integrated role of the cardiovascular system

Consisting of the heart and blood vessels, the cardiovascular system interacts with everything in your body. Your heart pumps red and white blood cells, proteins, minerals, platelets and hormones through your body. Your arteries carry blood away from the heart; the veins carry it back to the heart. Before blood goes back to your heart via your veins, your kidneys filter it and take waste and excess potassium, sodium and other salts out; this waste product is then taken out of the body through your urine. Your spleen filters out old red blood cells and clears bacteria from the blood.

The cardiovascular system is constantly at work delivering oxygen and nutrients to virtually all our body's cells and removing carbon dioxide and waste from them. Your fabulous heart supplies oxygenated blood to your body and your wonderful lungs pump blood back to your heart. The veins that carry blood to your heart are not as thick or elastic as the arteries that carry blood from your heart; muscular movement and gravity therefore assist the movement of blood back towards the heart, especially in poses where the legs or arms are raised higher than the heart.

Yoga can help to exercise the cardiovascular system,[40,41,42] and after some dynamic exercises you might be aware of your heart beating faster. Yoga can also help to slow the heart rate and lower blood pressure, helping the body to calm and relax.

The musculoskeletal system's role in the immune system

Moving the physical body also stimulates the musculoskeletal system, consisting of fascia, ligaments, tendons, muscles and bones. This includes the spongy tissue found inside your bones (bone marrow) that produces the red blood cells that carry oxygen, the white blood cells that fight infection and the platelets that help your blood clot. The bone marrow is also where all cells of the immune system are created from a common starting cell called a stem cell.

Yoga helps to build strength in the muscles and bones, thereby stimulating this part of the immune system. Having stronger muscles and bones also makes it easier to move independently, which is an important component of having a good quality of life.

The respiratory system's role

Your respiratory system draws oxygen in and carbon dioxide out. The cells in your body need energy and you receive that energy through the air you breathe into your body. Respiratory muscles draw breath into your body. Primary breathing muscles like the diaphragm (75%), intercostals (between the ribs) and the abdominals, do most of the work. Secondary breathing muscles in the neck and chest, also known as auxiliary muscles, are smaller muscles that help us to breathe when we need to get more air into the body, for instance, when we are exercising, and our heart rate speeds up.

The importance of breathing through your nose

Your nose is a fabulous breathing organ that warms, filters and cleans the air you breathe. Air is drawn into your two nostrils and then swirled through nasal hairs and mucus which trap dust and microbes. The air then enters a chamber or turbinate where it is further swirled around, picking up moisture and nitric oxide. Nitric oxide is necessary to increase carbon dioxide in the blood which in turn releases oxygen. James Nestor comments: 'sinuses release a huge boost of nitric oxide, a molecule that plays an essential role in increasing circulation and delivering oxygen into cells… nasal breathing alone can boost nitric oxide sixfold which is one of the reasons we can absorb about 18% more oxygen.'[43]

The nose also slows and deepens the breath and, as a result, the lungs fill more effectively from top to bottom. The mucus in our lungs traps foreign particles, and small hairs move this mucus upwards. Then, when we cough, we expel these foreign particles out of the body. The respiratory system is therefore a vital part of the immune system in its constant work defending against airborne invaders.

The nervous system's role in the immune system

Your nervous system is constantly feeding information back to your brain and it makes constant adjustments to your heart rate and blood pressure. Your brain communicates with your body via the central and peripheral nervous system. We have already looked at the longest cranial nerve, the vagus nerve (page 39), but we also have 31 pairs of peripheral spinal nerves that emerge from the spinal cord through the spaces between the vertebrae to connect internal organs and the musculoskeletal system of muscles, bones and joints. Nerves can be compressed by scar tissue and tight muscles which limit the body's range of motion. If nerves get affected and behave abnormally this is known as 'peripheral neuropathy' ('pathy' means abnormal); hands and feet can be affected, and this can make you feel less steady on your feet or unable to do small movements with your hands. By keeping your body supple and increasing your range of motion, you can help the functioning of your nerves and also help to keep your muscle strength if peripheral neuropathy is preventing you using your hands and/or feet fully. Muscles create not only bodily movements but also internal movements such as the eyes focusing, the heart beating and the movement of food through the intestines. Muscles cannot function without the nervous system to stimulate their activities.

The role of the digestive system

Whether your digestive system is working fully or not, you will be very aware of it and its ability to communicate its status. When we need food we feel hungry and sometimes our tummy growls; it may gurgle and make sounds as we digest; we feel thirsty when we haven't drunk enough water; and we will have wind and bowel movements. Sometimes we don't have bowel movements (constipation), or we have too many (diarrhoea); either can indicate that something is wrong in the our gut. This may involve the digestive part of our gut where proteins, fats and carbohydrates are broken down with the help of many enzymes, or the fermenting large bowel that is home to perhaps 10 trillion beneficial microbes that help to turn fibre into short-chain fatty acids. Collectively these are known has our 'microbiome' and they play a key part in our nervous and immune systems.

The gut has a semi-independent nervous system known as the 'enteric nervous system'. It is in constant communication with our brain and contains five times as many neurons as there are in our spinal cord. In addition, 90% of the feel-good hormone and neurotransmitter serotonin is produced in the gut;[44] the whole system helps to regulate our mood.

Working with it, our gut lining is (along with our skin) the key barrier between internal and external worlds and 80% of our immune system is associated with our gut. Our microbiome is key to its functioning and research shows that it can affect autoimmune-related diseases;[45] a huge part of our immunity comes from our gut.[46] The digestive system will eject pathogens from the body if we eat something that has 'gone off' and its mucus lining contains antibodies that work with the acid of the stomach to kill most microbes.

If you are recovering from an illness, then improving your gut microbiome is a crucial factor in allowing your body to repair itself. Furthermore, when you want to activate your immune system, your gut microbiome is essential for optimising immune surveillance.

How yoga can help the digestive system

When the sympathetic side of our nervous system is dominant (that is, when we are in fight-or-flight mode), there is less energy for digestion and a decrease in blood supply to the gut. When we stimulate the parasympathetic side of the nervous system, as we do in yoga, we know that this can help us with digestion. Poses that bring blood flow into the tummy area, help stretch it out and generally stimulate it, will also be really helpful for the digestive system. As this is a key part of repairing, you can follow sequences that focus on and support the downward movement of energy in elimination, which aids our digestion. According to Cancer Research UK: 'Being active helps move food through our bodies faster. This means anything harmful in food waste spends less time in our bowel, which may help to prevent bowel cancer.'[47]

The role of the lymphatic system

Our lymphatic system is the part of our immune system that deals with infections, cleanses tissues and maintains a balance of fluids in our body.[48] It circulates a protein-rich colourless fluid called lymph throughout our body; the lymph collects bacteria, viruses and waste and flushes them out. It is a one-way system, meaning that it goes in only one direction, from the periphery of the body (fingers and toes, arms and legs) back towards the centre of the body, draining into the bloodstream under our collarbones. The lymphatic system is made up of:

- **Lymph nodes** (also called lymph glands) that are found in clusters in the neck, abdome, chest, armpits and groin; these filter and clean the lymph, trapping bacteria and waste and destroying old and abnormal cells. Lymph nodes are tissues full of immune cells and they help to fight infection. We experience a sensation of 'swollen glands' as these nodes become enlarged with an expansion of immune cells when the body is fighting infection. Moving the body and opening and closing joints helps to encourage movement around the lymph nodes.
- **Lymph vessels** or tubes close to the surface of the skin carry the lymph that bathes our body's tissues and contains infection-fighting white blood cells. Like veins, these vessels have thin walls and carry the lymph at low pressure. They also have valves to prevent the back flow of lymph. As they are close to the surface of the skin they can be stimulated when we stretch.
- **White blood cells** or lymphocytes are the main type of blood cell found in the lymph; they include natural killer cells (or maybe if we change the language away from battling, these are also natural healing cells), T cells and B cells.

Once lymph has passed through the nodes it drains back into large veins behind the collarbones and then travels in the blood back to the heart and on to the kidneys where the blood is filtered, waste is removed and then excreted in our urine.

Lymph node removal and damage in cancer treatment

Lymph nodes may have been removed during treatment for cancer to check for cancer cells. A sentinel lymph node is the first lymph node that cancer is likely to spread to and so is the first to be removed for checking; this procedure is known as 'sentinel lymph node biopsy'. If cancer cells are detected in the sentinel lymph node then further lymph nodes may be removed. If the lymph nodes removed are in the armpit, or axilla, this is called 'axillary lymph node dissection' or 'clearance' and if they are in the groin, or inguinal nodes, then it is called 'inguinal node clearance'. Lymph node clearance is when most or all lymph nodes are removed.

Removal of lymph nodes and radiotherapy treatment that damages lymph nodes can prevent the lymphatic system working fully, and swelling known as lymphoedema can occur, often in the arms and legs. The removal of lymph nodes leads to the equivalent of a 'dead end' where there is no node for the lymph to flow into. However, there is research that shows that the clever lymphatic system can re-route after surgery to remove lymph nodes and find other pathways.[49, 50, 51] This is further evidence that the body is constantly at work to repair and heal.

How yoga can boost the lymphatic system

In yoga we can help boost the movement of the lymphatic system and give our body a helping hand by:

- **Breathing.** The main lymphatic vessel is the thoracic duct that runs through the diaphragm. If we are breathing fully the movement of the diaphragm massages the thoracic duct, moving lymph back up towards the heart.
- **Movement.** If we don't move, then our body can become sluggish. Movement encourages blood flow through the arteries and veins which run parallel to the lymph vessels and these therefore get stimulated as well.
- **Natural pump of muscles.** This is especially important in the muscles in the periphery of the body, like the calf muscles. Blood is pumped to our legs from the heart via arteries. When we compress our lower leg veins through contraction and relaxation of the calf muscles it helps to pump blood back

up the legs against gravity. As mentioned above, veins and lymph vessels, unlike arteries, don't have smooth muscle contractions to help push blood back to the heart; they have one-way valves that prevent the blood flowing backwards which is why, if we stand for too long, fluid pools in our lower legs and we get swelling around the ankles.

- **Stretching the skin.** When we stretch our muscles, we also stretch our skin which can stimulate the lymphatic vessels close to the surface of our skin. We can also stimulate our skin by gentle stroking.
- **Gravity.** In yoga we can position the body so that gravity can aid the movement of lymph towards the heart. If we elevate our legs or arms higher than our heart, gravity will be working in our favour to help move fluid back towards the heart.
- **Releasing scar tissue.** The lymph vessels are embedded in the fascia (the layer of connective tissue that surrounds all our organs and lines our body cavities) and if the fascia gets tight and restrictive it can act like a gate for the lymphatic system, preventing the free flow of fluids through the body. The more we can use yoga to create space around the tissues and release any stickiness in the fascia, the more circulatory flow we will create. The blood and the nerves share similar compartments, or 'neurovascular bundles', which we have on the inner edges of our thighs and pelvis and around our neck, shoulders and collarbone. Lots of practices in this book focus on creating space around the groin and armpit areas to ease any restrictions in the physical and energetic body.

If you have had lymph nodes removed then sequences for lubrication and flow will support the natural movement of the lymphatic system. Look for 5-minute practices for the lymphatic system labelled ⓛ.

If there is a risk of lymphoedema, then you will want to take time to build back strength slowly. My previous book, *Yoga for Cancer*, has more information on working with lymphoedema.

Yoga and the immune system

Our body was designed to move and there is evidence that being active does boost our immune system, making it work more effectively.[52] Yoga views the body as a whole, so to repair and strengthen the immune system means helping all these different systems work in union with each other.

7

The immune system and stress

Chronic and acute stress

Stress is an essential survival function for any living being and when our stress response is activated it empowers us to fight a potential threat or, if we are able, to run from that threat. If we are unable to escape then we might freeze and disconnect from the experience as our way of survival. Our stress can be an immediate reaction to a threat, known as acute stress, or it can be ongoing, in which case it is known as chronic stress.

When faced with a threat, our body releases the stress hormones adrenaline and cortisol to help us to defend ourselves (fight) or run away (flee). Their many effects include diverting blood supply away from organs not required in an emergency, such as the gut, towards the heart and respiratory system. Once we have defended ourselves or escaped, then those hormone levels go back to normal and the other systems affected resume their normal activities. However, if our stress is chronic then there will be an excessive and prolonged release of the stress hormones; levels stay elevated and other systems in the body are affected, including the immune system, with a decrease in natural killer cells. Natural killer cells are a type of lymphocyte (white blood cell) that are in the frontline of the immune system's defences against foreign invaders, infected cells and potential cancer cells. If we change the language around to healing, then these are the ultimate healing cells in the body. We know that natural killer cell activity is reduced in people with chronic stress, making them more open to infection, illness and cancer.

To fully understand how stress can affect the immune system we need to explore the nervous system further, and how it affects our immunity.

The autonomic nervous system

We divide our nervous system into the central nervous system (brain and spinal cord) and the peripheral nervous system. A component of the peripheral nervous system that regulates our heart rate, blood pressure, digestion, sexual arousal and respiration is the autonomic nervous system. It is made up of a network of nerves that handle the essential and unconscious body functions listed above. There are then three anatomical divisions to the autonomic nervous system known as the sympathetic, parasympathetic and enteric (gut) nervous systems. (The enteric nervous system was discussed in Chapter 6, page 44.)

The sympathetic nervous system

The sympathetic nervous system is our ON switch, activated any time we need to be active, get out of bed and on with our day. Located in the thoracic spine (the largest part of our spine where our ribcage is), it manages our heartbeat by regulating blood flow and it brings the energy of fight-or-flight as discussed above. When our sympathetic nervous system is stimulated, our heart beats faster and, in extreme situations where there is a threat or danger, our blood pressure increases significantly to get blood (oxygen and nutrients) to our vital organs, enabling us to run or stay and fight to protect ourselves.

As discussed above, when we feel scared or anxious our body releases stress hormones like adrenaline and cortisol. Adrenaline increases our blood pressure and boosts our energy; cortisol increases glucose (sugar) levels in our bloodstream and suppresses non-essential (in a fight-or-flight situation) systems in the body, including the immune system.[53] Another body system that stops functioning fully when this happens is the digestive system as it is not necessary to be digesting a meal if you need to run or fight. In extremely stressful situations you might vomit or lose control of your bowels or bladder. This may also explain why you might feel the need to urinate more frequently when you are waiting for test results or have 'scanxiety'[54] when waiting for scans and the results of scans.

If our stress is acute and not continuous, as with chronic stress, then once the stressful situation has ended our blood pressure and heart rate decrease and digestive and immune activity increase.

The parasympathetic nervous system

The parasympathetic nervous system is our OFF switch, putting us into what is known as 'rest-and-digest' mode. This is when healing and repair can take place and our immune system can function optimally.

The network of nerves that makes up the parasympathetic nervous system relaxes our body after periods of perceived danger or threat. However, to fully understand the impact of traumatic events we need to explore its two parts, as discovered by the distinguished scientist Stephen Porges.[55] By analysing research on the autonomic nervous system and the vagus nerve specifically, he discovered the ventral and dorsal parts of the vagus nerve.

The **ventral vagus system** is associated with feeling safe and connected and with our body functioning fully and able to repair. The **dorsal vagus system**, on the other hand, is activated when we are in grave danger and are unable to fight or flee and instead experience a freeze response. A surge in dorsal activity can result in a system shut-down: our heart rate and blood pressure drop, we go into shock and our body is flooded with endorphins. This is a primitive response that gives us animals a chance to survive an attack by a predator that might mistake us for dead and leave us alone. Many animals are wary of prey that is dead in case it might have gone off and eating it might make them ill. This may just create enough delay for us to escape an attack or, if not, the flood of endorphins will be a natural pain killer. It may also explain stories of people being able to run away from a situation only then to realise they are badly injured, but they hadn't felt any pain. In a traumatic situation people may disconnect or 'leave' their body. When this dorsal vagus part of the nervous system is dominant, you might experience feeling numb or disconnected – a sense of 'being here but not actually here', with everything slowing down so you have just enough energy to survive whilst going through the motions as if the experience wasn't happening to you. Some people describe a feeling of disconnection during a traumatic event where they were able to detach from themselves and view themselves as if the experience wasn't actually happening to them but they were witnessing it happening to someone else.

Being stuck in the sympathetic state where you constantly feel stressed, or being stuck in the dorsal, shut-down state feeling that you are unable to engage with the world around you, is an exhausting place to be mentally and physically and, as described, can be detrimental for your immunity and ability to repair. We can, however, stimulate the ventral vagus nerve anytime we slow down our exhale –

see chanting Aum (page 195) and Brahmari breathing (page 196) for lengthening exhales to calm the body and mind.

Recovering from trauma

Some quiet practices or body scans can feel traumatic if you do not feel safe being in your body as it triggers the dorsal vagus nerve. If this is the case, you may need to calmly activate your body to get back into the ventral vagus nervous system. In Bessel Van Der Kolk's excellent book *The Body Keeps the Score*,[56] he expands on Peter Levine's observation that we need to establish *islands of safety* in the body that are outside the reach of the dorsal vagus nerve. Areas like the hands and feet might allow you to ground and anchor in your own body to create a sense of being in control, present and fully alive. You will be able to heal and recover from trauma and, if you are experiencing chronic stress, despair or depression, you do not need to continue feeling like this; speak to your GP or seek support from a charity such as Mind.[57]

Our body is built to experience stress and react to stressful events. Acute stress is short-lived; chronic stress is ongoing, without any release or relaxation between challenges. We know that long-term activation of the sympathetic nervous system can disrupt our body's natural processes, which can increase our risk of health problems not only by suppressing the immune system but by promoting inflammation, elevating blood pressure and increasing blood clotting, raising the risk of heart attacks or strokes and creating feelings of anxiety and depression. Chronic stress also affects our digestive system, thins our bones and disrupts our sleep.

Learning some tools to help us deal with stress can improve our quality of life, lower our blood pressure and heart rate and increase our digestion as well as our immune system's ability to function fully; it can give us a sense of peace, even if the world around us does not feel peaceful. Being fully present also gives us time to move from doing to being, from a sense of dis-ease to being at-ease, from discomfort to balance. It allows us to respond to the situations around us rather than reacting and we might just start to feel that sense of connection and compassion to ourselves and others. Look for 5-minute practices labelled Ⓒ that are calming.

Smile, and the world smiles with you[58]

Mirror neurons are brain cells that allow us to mirror other people's expressions; this means that if someone smiles, we respond by smiling. These mirror neurons work faster than our conscious mind so the zygomaticus major muscles (from cheek bones to corners of the mouth) responsible for smiling will work even if we are told not to smile. These muscles respond first and start to mirror a smile, turning up the corners of our mouth, even if we consciously then decide to frown.

Smiling makes us feel good. Try it yourself. Turn up the corners of your mouth and notice how it makes you feel. Then try just having the essence of a smile by imagining you are smiling from the inside without the actual physical muscles working. The corners of your mouth don't actually turn up, but you just sense a smile shining out of your eyes like sunshine. How does this make you feel? Can you sense your body receiving that smile and maybe a sense of contentment growing from inside out? If it makes you feel good then you might just be confirming the research that suggests that smiling reduces cortisol and adrenaline levels. A happy face triggers specific chemical messengers like serotonin and endorphins. Serotonin helps to lift our mood and endorphins are a natural pain reliever and stress reducer; as a result, these are both known as happy hormones. Studies also show that endorphins help to heal damaged cells by increasing the immune cell activity around them and by decreasing inflammation.[59] Dopamine, another hormone that is released through smiling, activates the immune and digestive systems.

If we have the ability to mirror other people's expressions, then smiling is contagious; it is hard not to smile when we see someone genuinely smile and it makes us feel good when we smile. If we smile at other people we might just be contributing, one person at a time, one smile at a time, to making the world a better place. Maybe that person might feel good about themselves, and it might lead to them smiling at someone else, who might respond by feeling good and smiling at someone else? We may feel as though we aren't able to make huge changes in the world, but we can always start small, one person at a time. At triyoga where I teach, there is a sign on the wall that says, 'If you think you are too small to make a difference, try sleeping with a mosquito', which is widely attributed to the Dalai Lama. You never know the difference you might make to someone else's life just by smiling. This small movement of the zygomaticus major muscle might make a huge difference to someone's day, make them feel noticed or that they mattered, and they might pass this feeling on to someone else. How marvellous would that be and how good does it feel to think that you also are not too small to make a difference and, unlike the mosquito, without leaving an itchy bite?!

8

Building strength, bones and muscles

Our bones are living tissue that is constantly being remodelled. Bone is made up of living cells, such as osteoblasts that build bone and osteoclasts that remove older worn-out bone, embedded in a matrix of connective tissue. When we are young the osteoblasts work faster and our bones grow. As we get older the balance between osteoblasts and osteoclasts changes and more bone tissue may be removed than is built, which can lead to a weakening of our bones. Weight-bearing exercise is known to counteract this, as is the pull of our muscles on our bones (see more below).

Periods of inactivity, such as time in hospital or recovering from illness, can weaken our muscles and we can lose muscle mass. Strong muscles protect our joints as they take some of the pressure and weight off them. They also maintain our ability to do simple daily activities like walking upstairs, getting out of a chair unaided or carrying our shopping home from the supermarket. Our muscles attach via tendons and ligaments to our bones and when they are being stretched, as in yoga, they pull on our bones, stimulating the osteoblasts to build more bone.

Periods of inactivity due to illness or surgery can also lead to a loss of bone strength, as well as muscle mass. Studies have shown that yoga can reverse bone loss[60] even when it has reached the stage of osteoporosis. We start to lose bone mass from the age of 35[61] and women are more at risk of developing osteoporosis than men because of the part the hormone oestrogen plays in maintaining healthy bones. When women reach menopause and oestrogen levels drop, this can lead to a reduction in bone mass and as a result an increase in bone fragility and risk of fracture.[62]

Bending and twisting safely

According to the International Osteoporosis Foundation, forward bends and twists can increase the risk of spinal fractures;[63] however, if we are skilful in the way we practise, focusing on quality and not quantity, we can make our yoga practices safe even when bones are fragile. We need these movements in our daily life and don't want to stop twisting or forward bending; we just want to learn how to do these movements with the least risk of fracture.

The spine has more mobility for forward bending than backward bending and, as a result, it is more vulnerable to injury in forward-folds. Forward-bends put more pressure on the front of the vertebrae and increase the risk of compression or fracture here. The back of each vertebra has little facet joints that support us when we bend backwards.

If you think about your daily activities, we also forward-fold more in our daily lives than we back-bend; we need to forward-fold to get dressed, tie shoe laces and pick up objects from the ground, but we rarely bend backwards.

When forward-folding, try bending your knees so that your fold is at the top of your thighs – that is, hip flexion as opposed to spinal flexion. If you fold where your thighs meet your pelvis, then you can keep your spine neutral as you fold forward. This helps to prevent the rounding of your spine as you fold.

When we are twisting or rotating, we want to avoid rotating with any force so it is important to avoid using our limbs as levers to jam ourselves into deep rotations. Rather, we want to use our breath and the deeper muscles of our core to help us to rotate. Try exhaling fully making a 'ssshh' sound until all the breath has left your body. Can you feel your core engaging? We want to use these muscles to rotate us to one side. Always find length first, so breathe in and grow tall, thereby creating some space between your vertebrae. Then keep that length as you exhale and use your breath (and core) to rotate you to one side. Once you are in the twist, then your arms and legs can help you to stay in the pose but should not be used to force more twisting. As you exhale feel your core muscles turning you to one side so you are letting your breathing do the work of deepening the pose as you exhale. That way the rotation comes from within your body.

If you are at risk of osteoporosis, then practise forward-folding and rotating in the safe way described above, and following the sequences in this book will help you move in a way that encourages bone strength without increasing the risk of fractures.

Yoga is fantastic at putting weight on different parts of the body and moving the body in different planes which can help to improve bone quality, balance and resilience.

A key component of moving safely is keeping the natural curves of our spine, often referred to as the neutral curves (see Figure 4a on page 61). According to Andrew McGonigle, the natural curves in our spine 'make the structure particularly stable, allowing for the distribution of body weight and the absorption of shock, helping with balance and facilitating movement'.[64]

When you are stretching muscles, you should feel a healthy stretch in the belly or middle of the muscle away from the tendons and ligaments that are close to the joint. If you are feeling any sensations close to the joint that are sharp, throbbing or stabbing, then you need to ease out of the stretch to see if that releases the sensation. If it does not, then you should come out of the pose. You might feel the sensation of muscles working and maybe those same muscles fatiguing, but you should not experience any discomfort in the joints of the knees, hips, shoulders or elbows.

Improving balance

Weakness in muscles and stiffness in joints can also make balancing more challenging as we can't move easily from one position to another. Our senses feed information back to our brain about the environment around us and the potential hazards as we move about our day. Uneven surfaces, distracting noises, busy, bustling environments and strong winds are all things that can make moving around more difficult and the risk of falling greater. We aren't as connected to the earth beneath us as our ancestors would have been because we wear shoes; our foot then works as one unit and we don't use the small bones in our feet to adjust to any uneven terrain. Most of our surfaces are flat and so our feet don't get a chance to move fully, feel the changing ground beneath us and learn to adapt to it. Yoga does give us the opportunity to be barefooted, as we practise yoga with our shoes off. This gives us a chance to actually feel the ground beneath us, the texture of the mat or floor under our feet and to fully feel the connection of our feet to the earth beneath us. If you add to that a quietening of the mind and a focus on breathing and the present moment, you might find with practice your balance improves.

I find in my own yoga practice that I am more likely to fall out of my balancing poses when I get distracted and my mind wanders. If I'm not in the present moment and I am mindless (i.e. my mind is elsewhere), instead of being mindful, then I lose balance. I think this is often the case when something happens to make us fall – we are in a hurry and not being mindful of where we are going and the potential obstructions. We are much more likely to fall when we are distracted and don't notice an uneven pavement or an obstacle in our way and trip. It is interesting that by keeping the body supple, our reflexes are quicker and if we do stumble or trip we can adjust to the movement, respond to our fall and be less likely to hurt ourselves. Keeping flexible can make the difference between catching ourselves from falling and actually falling and potentially hurting ourselves.

This is particularly important as we get older because the most serious consequence of falling in older people is hip fracture. Hip fractures and the complex medical and rehabilitation needs post-surgery are associated with loss of independence and increased mortality rates.[65] Some studies suggest that hip fractures lead to an increased mortality of 30% after one year[66] which means one in three adults over the age of 65 dies within 12 months of a hip fracture.

Osteoporosis (see above) is often called the 'silent' disease because bone loss can occur with no symptoms until you experience a fall, break or fracture. It is very important therefore to build bone strength, to move in ways that are safe and to learn to improve balance. Balance is a skill we can learn and re-learn at any age and this is also true of building bone and muscles. Just practise without judgment or frustration, which is sometimes the biggest challenge. The practices in Chapters 14 and 16 that help with building strength have the symbol ⑤.

Movement and static postures

'Motion is lotion' – in other words, movement helps to lubricate the joints. Just like oiling the hinges of a door to stop it creaking, movement lubricates your body's joints. It is very common to hear noises when you move your joints – known as crepitations. If you are not experiencing any pain with these sounds, then there is no need to be concerned as it is perfectly normal. However, if pain is accompanying the sounds, then you might want to get some further advice from a professional.

Often the sequences in this book involve dynamic movements, where you warm up the joints by moving in and out of poses, to prepare the body for static postures or poses which you might hold for a few breaths. Static postures can be more demanding physically and can also be challenging if you are recovering from trauma or surgery, so you may prefer to stay quite dynamic with the postures, moving in and out of poses instead of holding them for a few breaths.

When holding static postures, we can work on activating the opposing muscles to the ones that are being stretched. Each muscle in the body is paired with an opposing muscle (together these are called agonist-antagonist pairs); when the agonist contracts the antagonist relaxes. So, for example, if we engage our quadriceps (the muscle at the front of the thigh) by gently hugging the muscle to the bone and firming the muscles around our knee by lifting the kneecap up, this will help the back of the thigh (hamstring) release. In this example the quadriceps is the agonist and the hamstring is the antagonist. This process is known as reciprocal inhibition and prevents muscles working against each other. Engaging muscles also helps to support the joints by creating stability there and also by giving us some space around the joint.

A joint is a meeting of bones, cartilage, synovial fluid, ligaments, tendons and muscles. We want to reduce wear and tear in the joints and, by engaging the muscles that surround a particular joint, we can help to lift the bones away from each other and give some space at the joint. It is important when balancing that we don't 'sit' into a joint – that we use our muscles, by firming them, to support it and create space in it, thereby avoiding wear and tear on the cartilage that surrounds the articulating surfaces. This helps to protect the tendons, ligaments and cartilage so they aren't over-worked or worn away.

When standing normally, notice how you stand. Do you feel even on your two feet? Do you stand by collapsing over to one side? (See Figure 4 as an example of how we often stand.) Do you lock your knees? Can you create a micro-bend in your knees so that your leg looks straight even when you know it isn't fully straight? Then see if you can keep that and engage the quadriceps muscles at the front of your thighs to support your knees.

Some poses can be challenging to the joints. If the joints are being compressed and you feel pinching sensations this also might be a sign that you have gone too far into a pose. This could result in a numbing or tingling feeling in your extremities as the compression puts pressure on blood vessels and nerves. You might need to back off out of the stretch and experiment with using yoga props (see page 69) to help to create some space in your joints. Look out for the (J) to indicate poses that involve the joints.

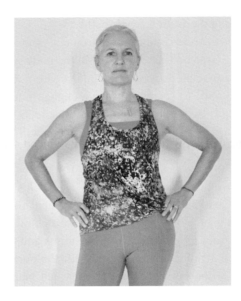

Figure 4 Hanging out in the joints

Start small and build up

When recovering from an illness or surgery it is a good idea to start small and build back strength slowly. When balancing, use the support of props like chairs or walls. If you haven't been able to practise for a while or you are currently going through treatment for cancer, then you might not be building strength but just maintaining muscle strength and keeping a range of motion (ROM). If you have recently had surgery, please do ask your surgeon if there is anything you should not do or if there is a limit to range of motion in a certain direction that you should be aware of.

All of the practices in this book can be done on their own, but you can also lengthen them or make them more challenging by increasing the repetition of dynamic poses and increasing the time you hold a static pose. You can also add various sequences together to make a longer practice. To make it easier, you can rest in-between poses, or have fewer repetitions of dynamic poses or hold static poses for a shorter period of time. With this book you really can customise your practice to fit your needs in any given moment.

Rest

It is also really important to highlight here the value of rest and restorative yoga to help strengthen your bones. When we are stressed, and those stress levels stay elevated, we produce higher levels of cortisol which can prevent the deposition of calcium and minerals in the bones. Cortisol also triggers bone mineral resorption (removal) to free up amino acids (the protein that forms the underlying matrix of bone) for use as an energy source.[67] Bone cell growth is consequently reduced and the bone remodelling that occurs throughout life is disrupted. Any practices that bring us into the 'rest and digest' side of our nervous system are calming or soothing and are going to help to reduce levels of cortisol.[68] Look for practices labelled Ⓒ that are calming.

The natural curves of your spine

As mentioned above, our spine has natural curves which allow it to be strong and support the weight of our body but also provide flexibility and movement. As illustrated in Figure 4a, we have a concave curve in our cervical (neck) spine which has seven vertebrae, a convex curve in our thoracic (rib cage) spine which has 14 vertebrae and a concave curve in our lumbar spine (lower back) which has five vertebrae. The sacrum and coccyx (our tailbone) make up the rest of the spine and have a convex curve too.

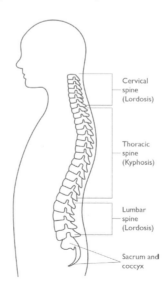

Cervical
spine
(Lordosis)

Thoracic
spine
(Kyphosis)

Lumbar
spine
(Lordosis)

Sacrum and
coccyx

Figure 4a Natural curves
of the spine

The spine contains the spinal cord which is like a highway for information between the organs and muscles and the brain. Fluid around the brain and spinal cord is known as cerebrospinal fluid; it provides the nerve tissue of the spinal cord and brain with nutrition and oxygen and helps to remove waste materials. It also provides lubrication between the surrounding bones and the spinal cord. Good posture helps to maintain a healthy spine, and poor posture can stress the spinal column and restrict the movement of fluids, including blood flow. In this book we also look at how poor posture limits the movement of the diaphragm and reduces space for the digestive system (see Chapter 5).

Keeping the natural curves of your spine will also affect how you feel energetically. You can try yourself by observing what it feels like if you slump your body, round your spine and collapse your chest. Notice how much harder it is to get breath and energy into your body when the front of the body closes. You might even feel a slump in energy as you restrict the movement of breath and prana into your body. Now try sitting on your sitting bones, as opposed to your tailbone, and lengthen your spine so you grow taller. Lengthen up through the crown of your head, without lifting your chin, and gently guide your shoulder blades down your back so you feel your chest opening. Now observe how this feels. Is it easier to breathe?

To explore what a natural or neutral spine actually feels like:

- Lie on your back. Bend your knees and place your feet about as wide apart as your hips; try moving your feet outwards and inwards to find a comfortable position. Then move your feet towards your bottom and away from it to find a place that feels most comfortable to you.
- Bring your awareness to your sacrum, coccyx and lumbar spine. Your sacrum is the large triangular bone that fits into your pelvis above the crease of your bottom. Your tailbone or coccyx attaches to the bottom of your spine. When you lie on the floor most of the weight of your pelvis will be on your sacrum.
- Breathe in gently, letting your pubic bone move away from your head.
- As you exhale, draw your pubic bone towards your head. Feel how your lower back presses into the mat (flexion) (see Figure 5a).
- Inhale, feel your pubic bone move away from you and how you get some space at your lower back (lumbar) (see Figure 5b).
- Exhale, and feel your pubic bone move towards you and how your lower back rounds towards the floor.

These small movements of pelvic rocking can help bring movement and breath into the pelvis but also make us aware of how our spine can round (flexion) towards the mat or curve away from the mat (extension). A neutral spine is somewhere in the middle (see Figure 5c).

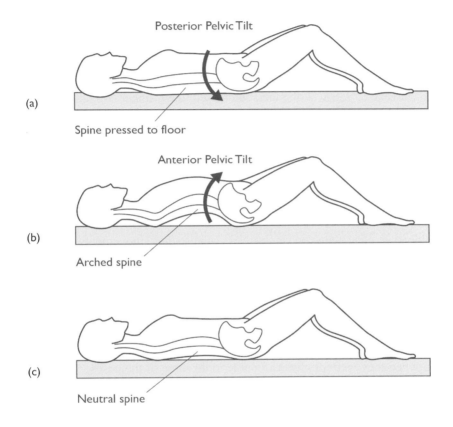

Posterior Pelvic Tilt

(a)

Spine pressed to floor

Anterior Pelvic Tilt

(b)

Arched spine

(c)

Neutral spine

Figure 5 Finding natural curves of spine a) posterior tilt; b) anterior tilt; c) neutral spine

Natural curves of the spine or a 'neutral spine' describes when the spine feels long and not rounded or flattened. A neutral spine is something we will come back to throughout this book as it is a key component of practising yoga safely. When we are working with the natural curves of our spine it is stronger and we are able to incorporate the deep core muscles and use them to help support us.

Kinaesthetic imagery: visualising building strength

Our ability to imagine can have a powerful influence on how we feel. In my previous book, *Yoga for Cancer*, I explored how being compassionate or having kind thoughts had a positive influence on the body and the immune system. Many books have been written on how kindness and compassion help to boost our immune system and I highly recommend the work of Dr David Hamilton and Dr Dean Ornish.[69, 70]

It is also possible to use our mind to visualise moving our body not only to reduce loss of muscle mass[71] but also to become physically stronger. At the Lerner Institute in Cleveland, USA, volunteers increased their finger strength by 35% through visualising extending and contracting their little finger.[72] Other studies using visualisation found muscle strength increased significantly. The more vividly the subjects who participated in the study imagined contracting muscles, the more strength they gained.[73] Furthermore, the more effort that was put into the visualisation, the stronger the results.[74]

These techniques have been used by stroke patients to help to train their brain circuits and build strength in the physical body. This means that if there are days when you are unable to practise yoga you can instead visualise these movements happening. Visualise your muscles working as you read through the sequences (see page 183) and imagine raising your arms and legs or feeling muscles contracting as you imagine balancing or moving through poses. I have worked with many students who have had no choice but to work like this for a period of time. It can be a challenging practice, but I know that you can still experience the quieting quality of yoga even by simply visualising moving dynamically. It has allowed students still to be able to practise in a class even when they weren't physically able to do some of the poses, giving them access to the shared experience of participating with a supportive community. Now that many yoga classes have an online option, yoga is even more accessible. You can participate in a group class from the comfort of your own home. I have even had students come to class from the luxury of their beds and been able to fully participate in a yoga for cancer class.

9

Starting to practise

How much time do you realistically have available to practise yoga? Can you find 5 minutes? What do you feel you need from your practice today? Take a moment just to ask yourself, 'What support do I need right now?' Ask without judgment so that you truly start to explore what you need as opposed to what you think you *should* do. Your focus might be to support your digestive system by doing 5 minutes to aid digestion, or to stimulate the lymphatic system with 5 minutes to encourage lubrication and flow. Maybe you just need 5 minutes of calm or cooling. You are the only person who knows what it feels like to be you and therefore what will be supportive to you in this moment, and this will change from day to day. Some days you might not be sure what it is that your body needs so you could just try flicking through this book, opening a random page and seeing where the universe takes you. What 5-minute practice do you open up to?

Each 5-minute practice in the book has an associated symbol, and the previous chapters have introduced you to what the symbols mean. The list below summarises the six types of practice.

- (C) Calming
- (E) Energising
- (J) Lubricating joints
- (L) Lymphatic system
- (S) Strengthening muscles and bones

The sequences you decide to follow might also be determined by the space you have for your 5 minutes, or your location. It might be easier to do a 5-minute seated sequence, or even a supine (lying on your back) sequence that has been adapted for a chair such as 5-minutes for digestion (page 101), if you are at work. You may want a standing sequence if you have been seated for a long time and feel a bit stagnant.

The time of day may also impact your decision on what practice to do. You may have more energy at the beginning of a day for standing postures but by the end of the day feel that a restorative practice is going to be more beneficial for you. Little and often is the key to creating a habit that hopefully you will find makes you feel better than you did before you started.

Tailoring your practice

You can always build on this good feeling and you might find that you want to combine a few of the 5-minute practices, and explore how a combination works for you. You can do this by observing how you feel after you have practised. If you are wanting to combine some 5-minute practices, it is always good to start with something supine or seated and end with something more calming and soothing like a restorative practice or a breathing meditation practice; you might even sandwich some standing postures in-between these. You can be playful as you build onto your 5-minute practice, and if you have more time some days it could grow into a 10-minute, 15-minute or even longer practice. You become the creator of your yoga by trying out different combinations of 5-minute practices, and then noticing how it has made you feel at the end of the practice.

You can tailor your practices to suit your time, your energy levels or what you need in that moment. This, I think, is really crucial when taking back a sense of control and when healing – you get to decide what you want to practise, what your focus will be and how long you get to practise for.

I often ask at the beginning of my classes if anyone has any special requests and have found that releasing and opening the feet is popular, as is stimulating the lymphatic system, as it is part of the immune system and therefore really beneficial when recovering or repairing the body. So, if I were to ask you what your requests are today, what would you say? Drop your awareness down into your heart and ask yourself, 'What would I like to focus on today?' Just see what pops up into your heart. This could be a great way to start.

These practices are created so that they can be done by anyone living with cancer and this might also include living with a PICC line, stoma or port-a-cath. You need to be six-weeks post-surgery, with all surgical incisions healed.

The first thing you will need to practise is being kind. Being kind involves following the first limb of the eight-fold path of yoga[75] which is **ahimsa**. Ahimsa means non-harming and non-violence; wherever there is the absence of violence there is the presence of love. So, the first limb of yoga is to be kind. This means that being kind is doing yoga. Being kind to yourself means having some compassion when you have setbacks, can't find time or are unable to do something, rather than being unkind, harsh, critical and judgmental of yourself. In a physical sense this would be moving in a pain-free way and not pushing through pain. Also moving in a way that is kind to yourself and not seeing it as being 'wimpy' or thinking that you are not trying hard enough; instead accept that sometimes we need to start small and build slowly.

Some days we have more energy than others and some days we wake up and our body feels like a bag of glued-up cement! It is better to have a pain-free range of motion and build on that rather than do something that causes you to injure yourself and then puts you off yoga. Hopefully yoga is something you can do for life, so listen to the sensations: what does it actually feel like in your body? Pain is your body's way of telling you to back off, so start to notice these sometimes-small sensations in your body or the 'red flags' that pop up warning you that something isn't right. If you are ever in doubt, just leave a movement out or ease out of a pose. It can feel intense sometimes if you are working with areas of scar tissue or areas you have protected or guarded, but it shouldn't be painful, especially in the joints. We are always working to achieve pain-free motion and practising kindness.

Create an intention for your practice

When I first started yoga and heard a teacher say 'set an intention for your practice' I had absolutely no idea what they were talking about. I wasn't sure what kind of intention I was supposed to have and then I was worried that I didn't have the right kind of intention. An intention is another way of taking back some control and finding a focus for your practice – something that guides you through your practice, especially if it becomes difficult. It can be another way of anchoring into the present moment. In fact, staying present for the time that I am on my mat is often my intention, because staying present is sometimes the hardest part of my yoga practice. Maybe your focus or intention might be to stay with your breath for the full 5 minutes or to be grateful for your breath, or maybe there is something else that motivated you to get onto your mat and practise yoga? What was your purpose for practising or what is your desire for your practice? What do you need more of today? What helps you feel inspired to practise or is there something you would like to embody as you move?

Your intention might be something you come back to throughout your practice or throughout your day. Maybe you find it is motivating to have an intention or that the practice has greater meaning because it animates the practice and focuses it? Your intention may be different depending on the time of day you practise. A morning practice with the whole day ahead might require a different focus to an evening practice where your intention might be to let go of the day that has been and prepare for sleep. The same sequence or practice can have a different outcome if you set an intention or a focus for it and you can explore by observing how this feels and if this gives your practice more depth.

Create a safe space to repair

I find it is really helpful to create a special space to practise that is personal and can feel a little bit like a mini sanctuary – putting your phone on silent and moving away from the distractions of computers or work so that you signal to yourself that this is 'my time', time that you are taking out of your day to put yourself first. Is there a good time of day when you know you are less likely to be disturbed? Can you let people around you know that you are taking 5 minutes out for you?

When I first started to change my practice from something I did a couple of times a week to a daily practice, my children were still really small. One summer holiday I decided to negotiate with them. I told them that if they let me have my hour for *me*, then the rest of the day would be about *them*, but that Mum (me) just needed an hour to herself to practise her yoga (or 'yogamats' as my youngest called it). This was in hindsight probably quite unrealistic with three small children but nevertheless I rolled out my mat with them quietly playing with toys around me and started to practise yoga. Of course, this peace didn't last very long. After a few minutes there was some infighting and someone demanding my immediate attention. I got off my mat and lost my temper. All I had wanted was this one hour for me and I was cross that my children couldn't even give me that, but as I berated them I realised that, by losing my temper, I had lost all aspects of 'doing yoga'. There was no point in my being all calm and 'yogic' on my mat if the smallest thing rubbed me up the wrong way and pushed my buttons so that I became angry. It was a revelation to me: I was never going to find the promised enlightenment at the end of my yoga journey if I couldn't practise what I felt on the mat, off the mat.

I learnt to register the sounds around me but not let them create disturbances in my mind and body and that really my yoga practice was only going to benefit me in my life if I could use it to establish a calmness to all that was going on around me even if I didn't like whatever that was. It made me more interested in learning how to find an inner peace – a peace that could stay with me despite my chaotic external situation. The yogic texts told me that our true nature is inherently kind and peaceful, and this was something I wanted to work towards, on my mat and off. Donna Farhi in *Bringing Yoga to Life* says 'what greater enlightenment could we possibly attain than to become a decent person... the person who restores our faith in human nature... this fundamental goodness *is* our true nature'.[76]

We might not be able to find 5 minutes away from children and pets, so maybe they need to be incorporated into the practice and maybe part of the practice will be staying present even when the sounds around you are drawing you out of that moment. If you can stay steady, calm and non-judgmental during these moments then you are definitely doing yoga. If you viewed your reflection in water that was moving, you wouldn't see your true reflection. You would only see this when the water stopped moving, settled and became calm and not wavy. Same thing with yoga. When you quieten everything, you can get a glimpse of that true nature or reflection that is unchanging, unlike the space around you. My children eventually got used to me practising around them and often I could hear them whispering if one was noisy, 'Ssshhh, Mum's doing yogamats'.

Props

Speaking of yoga mats, a yoga mat can help provide some padding when we are lying on the floor for supine poses, but it also helps prevent us slipping when we are doing any standing postures. We also use yoga bricks to elevate the floor when it doesn't quite meet us or straps to lengthen our arms when they are just not long enough to reach something. These props are really useful to help make poses accessible, which is especially important when we might need to modify poses due to scar tissue, tight areas or other things like lymphoedema that can limit our range of motion or movement.

Throughout lockdown we modified using tin cans or dictionaries instead of blocks, and scarfs or belts instead of straps, so you can be creative in how you modify. However, if you find that yoga is helpful to you then it might be worth investing in a couple of bricks (brick-sized yoga blocks), a strap and a bolster. Bolsters are really useful in restorative poses and great for lying over to open up the chest and release tension. You can create a bolster yourself by rolling a pillow lengthways in a towel or blanket. If you are looking to purchase yoga equipment, then yogamatters.com has a great selection of yoga props (see Figure 6).

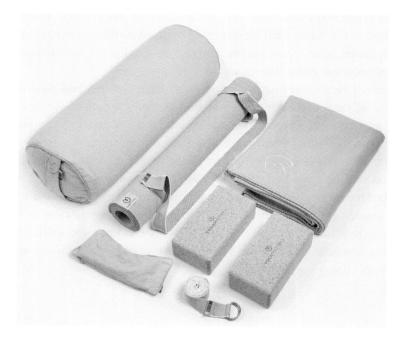

Figure 6 Props (Yogamatters)

Chair support

Alongside the practices in this book are some suggestions as to how the poses can be done with the support of a chair. There are a few reasons I have included the chair options:

1. There may be periods when getting down onto the floor or up from it are not possible. The chair gives you an option still to be able to practise yoga, as opposed to feeling that it is impractical and therefore not for you.

2. Using a chair may make the practices more accessible to you and easier for you to take the 5 minutes of time to create a habit that grows into a daily practice. If you are practising at your desk, see if you can turn off your computer or close down your laptop (see above about creating a safe space to practise). I think it helps to start by stopping whatever it is you were doing. Make a distinction between 'work' and 'me time'.

3. If balance is an issue, then you might want to use the chair as a support for standing postures, especially when building back strength after any periods of bed rest or inactivity. Again, it is better to start small and build up strength and confidence, so you don't feel frustrated with the practice.

4. Finally, there are many ways to do the same posture and there isn't a 'one-size fits all' so you can try the postures with the chair and without, to mix up your practice and to explore how the support of the chair feels.

I have also included some more challenging options with the chair for you to try and explore how these feel in your body. If you think the chair might slide when you are using it, then you can place it against the wall so that it doesn't move as you do.

71

Fig.13

10

Mudras – hand gestures

Some yoga practices are subtle and work on the energetic or breath body, as described in Chapter 12. I have included mudras as these can be done by anyone, at anytime and anywhere. Even if you have days in hospital or are too fatigued to move, then you can practise the hand gestures to explore the effects.

Mudra translates as 'to gesture' and can be by hand or eye or even ways that you sit (asana). In this book, we will be focusing on the hands. We are intuitive beings and often use our hands unconsciously to gesture something, like crossing fingers to wish someone good luck, or giving a thumbs up or clapping our hands to show appreciation. We also give a thumbs down to show we aren't so happy with something, and we can even use our fingers to create a gesture that may be considered offensive. Sometimes I think we intuitively place our fingers in a way to help us think – for example touching our fingers together like a tee pee to help us remember something. That gesture is said to stimulate the right and left hemispheres of the brain so it could be an aid in recollecting something. It is known as **hakini** mudra, see Figure 7.

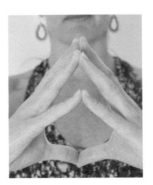

Figure 7 Hakini mudra

The placement of our hands can be really powerful and, if I feel disconnected or upset, I will often place the heel of my hand on the centre of my breastbone and my other hand over that hand; placing my hands like this on my heart gives me a sense of calm and grounding. I also use my fingers to tap under my collarbones to stimulate the stress receptors there (see Figure 8), and this I find incredibly calming.

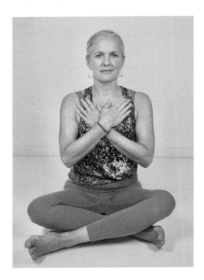

Figure 8 Tapping collar bones

So maybe you already naturally and intuitively do something with your hands to create a sense of calm or to help you concentrate, or maybe you will find a mudra in this book that you connect to.

There is no scientific evidence to support mudras, but our fingers give our brain information all the time. Through their nerves and connective tissue our hands tell us if a surface is hot or cold, rough or smooth. So, in reverse can we send messages of love or repair from our brain to our hands? It is definitely worth exploring, isn't it?

In reflexology, parts of the fingers and hands are connected to other areas of the body or internal organs. In Chinese medicine, stimulating the meridian lines in the fingers and hands can relieve a symptom somewhere else in the body. In Ayurveda, the fingers represent the elements: the thumb is fire, the index finger air, the middle finger ether, the ring finger earth and the little finger water.

Getting started

Before practising with mudras, it is often good to sit and just observe your breathing. Notice what your breath feels like? Notice where it is more dominant – front of body? Sides of body? Back of body? Does your breath get stuck anywhere? Can you breathe down into your belly? Is it easier to breathe down one side of your body? If you make these observations, when you do focus on your hands are you able to gauge if anything changes with your breath and, if so, do you notice what has changed?

Start by sensing where your fingers touch. Observe your breathing, again noticing if it is more challenging to breathe with the mudra. If it is more challenging to breathe, then I would release the mudra and try a different one.

Sometimes you can also direct your breath into your hands or another area of the body. Energy follows awareness. Try it yourself. Close your eyes and bring your awareness to your right hand. Notice what changes. Does it become warmer? Are you aware of movement of energy – swirling sensations in the palm or the palm feeling more zingy or energised?

Mudras that support prana

Ⓔ **Prana mudra** is said to activate the root chakra, grounding and anchoring, helping to increase energy and vitality. Place the tips of the thumb, ring and little fingers together. Keep the other fingers extended. They may not fully straighten but they should be extending rather than bending (see Figure 9).

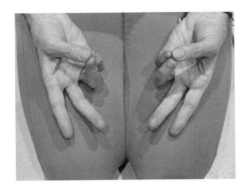

Figure 9 Prana mudra

Mudras that support apana

Ⓛ **Apana vayu mudra** helps with the downward movement of energy and the 'healing and strengthening of the heart'.[77] Bring the tips of the index fingers of both hands to touch the base of the thumbs. Then bring the tips of the middle and ring fingers to touch the tips of your thumbs (see Figure 10).

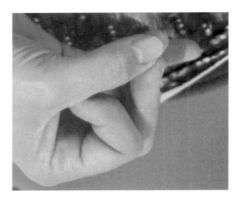

Figure 10 Apana vayu mudra

Mudras that support samana vayu

Ⓒ **Matangi mudra**: Interlace all of your fingers except the middle fingers. Extend your middle fingers and place them against each other. Then lower your hands to rest at your belly with your fingers pointing out away from your navel (see Figure 11).

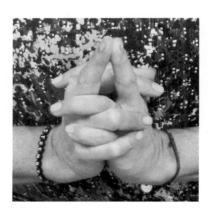

Figure 11 Matangi mudra

Mudras that support vyana

Ⓛ **Garuda mudra**, said to 'activate blood flow and circulation',[78] invigorates the organs and balances energy on both sides. Hook your thumbs and place your hands onto your belly with your right hand on top of your left (see Figure 12).

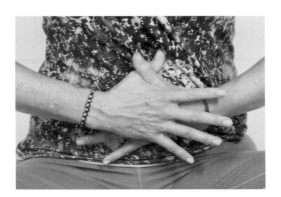

Figure 12 Garuda mudra

Ⓙ Ⓛ **Vajra mudra** is also said to stimulate circulation. With both hands extended out (see Figure 13), press your thumb to the side of the middle finger by the nail. Press the ring finger to the other side of the middle finger and the little finger at the side of your ring fingernail.

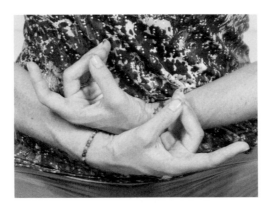

Figure 13 Vajra mudra

Mudras that support udana

ⓒ **Shankh mudra**: Close your left thumb into the fingers of your right hand and then bring your right thumb to the extended fingers of your left hand (see Figure 14). Create sounds and vibrations as you hold the hands against your sternum.

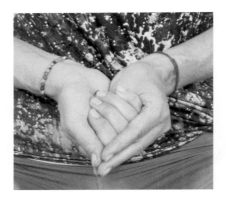

Figure 14 Shankh mudra

11

Mantras to anchor

If an elephant was allowed to roam through a market it could cause a lot of chaos with its trunk. It would eat things, throw things and be able to knock things over. Its trunk is like our mind. Left on its own it can cause a lot of destruction. However, if you give an elephant a stick to hold it will curl its trunk around the stick and proudly hold the stick as it moves through the market. With the trunk stilled by the stick it limits the amount of destruction it can cause. If our mind is a trunk, then the stick can be a mantra. Mantra translates as 'man' meaning mind and 'tra' meaning transcend or it can also mean tool, a tool for the mind or a help to transcend our thinking mind.

When we repeat a mantra, this is known as **japa**. Mantras are also described as tools to protect as in 'to protect us from our mind'. The philosopher and poet Mark Nepo, in his poem 'Coming up for air',[79] describes the mind as being 'like a spider, it will weave many webs' and he says we must 'be aware, mostly of ourselves' and so a mantra is not only a tool for our mind, but it also gives us protection from our mind.

Sanskrit words are said to be imbued with energy and as this energy is then transmitted to the body, mantras have traditionally been seen as healing. According to *Prana Vidya*,[80] 'the power of mantra affects prana which in turn heals the body and transforms the mind'. Traditionally, a mantra was given to you by a guru or enlightened spiritual teacher but there are some mantras that are considered universal, such as **aum**, **so ham** and the **gayatri mantra**. You can also explore how creating other sounds, like the root sounds associated with the chakras (page 24), or even plain and simple humming, create natural vibrations in our body that can calm or energise.

When you work with sounds or mantras, read the words, mentally forming the pronunciation in your head and let the word, words or sounds move throughout the whole of your body. Imagine infusing your cells with the sounds. There is evidence that even just listening to singing bowls and gongs helps to induce 'deep relaxation response and participants (in a 2017 study) reported significantly less tension, anger, fatigue and depressed mood'.[81]

We know that humming stimulates the parasympathetic side of the nervous system because the vocal cords contract to make the sound and this partial obstruction creates a vibration that soothes the nervous system. Studies also show that sound can help improve the tone of the vagus nerve.[82] Cats purr not just because they are happy but because the vibrations created when they purr help to calm and soothe their nervous system.

Throughout history, chanting has been used by tribes and communities to communicate devotion to higher powers, gods and nature, and to help with the healing of illnesses. Sound can create changes in energy and in mood and therefore make us feel better. The energetic vibrations of chanting mantras can help to energise, create prana or create peace. Sound works on the subtle energetic body which is linked to the physical body. Chanting activates energy and can help to clear stuck energy in the chakras or energetic body to help the body flow with ease.

The universal mantras

Aum

Aum is chanted to connect to the universe and tune into our higher sense of self. According to the ancient texts, aum is the seed word or **bija** that all words and sounds come from. Place a hand on your belly and one at the centre of your chest and take a breath in and chant the 'a' sound as in 'awe'. Notice where you feel any vibrations in your body or under your hands. Then, as you exhale, chant the 'u' sound as in 'oooh'. Then take a breath in and as you exhale chant 'mmm' and notice where you feel sensations and movements from the sound. Then try putting the sounds together: 'awe', 'oooh', 'mmm' so they make the sound 'aum'. Try also changing the tone of your chant to see if a lower tone resonates with you.

When you chant the 'awe', bring your awareness to the space between the base of your spine and the centre of your navel. As you move into the 'oooh' sound, bring awareness to the space between the navel centre and your throat. When you move into the 'mmm' sound, bring your awareness to the space between your throat and the crown of your head. Sense the vibrations at these various places along your spine.

Chanting aum helps to lengthen your exhale, which reduces feelings of being stressed by stimulating the parasympathetic side of the nervous system.

So ham

So ham is a mantra that mimics the subtle sound of the breath and translates as 'I am all that I need to be'. In *Moving Inwards: The Journey to Mediation,* Rolf Sovik explains that so ham (pronounced 'so hum') means 'That I am, the self… I am'.[83] The mantra is reminding us that the inner self stays the same no matter what our external situation is. In *Healing Mantras* by Thomas Ashley-Farrand, the mantra 'brings the mind in tune with the divine self within'.[84] I use this mantra often in class as an anchor into the present moment.

Inhale hearing the sound 'so' and exhale hearing the whisper of 'hum'. Repeat anytime you are having a thought as a way of coming back into the present moment. I know that I can easily 'think' my way through a yoga class, but breath and this mantra really do work to keep me present.

The gayatri mantra

The gayatri mantra is my favourite. It is an invocation to the sun and said to be one of the most auspicious mantras. It is the ultimate gratitude mantra, giving thanks to the sun that is forever giving and never receiving and asking that the light of the sun shines through all of us and inspires all of us and that in return we will go out, beaming light and gratitude to others and inspire and uplift those we come into contact with.

The syllables in the gayatri mantra (see the list) when chanted create a vibration in the energy channels of the body, awakening and opening, allowing energy to flow through this subtle body. Visualise the light of the sun beaming through your heart and out of your heart, sending light and love to everyone.

Om
Bhur Bhuvah Swaha
Tat Savitur Varenyam
Bhargo Devasya Dhimahi
Dhiyo Yo Nah Prachodayat.

A recording of the gayatri mantra can be found on my website at https://vickyfox-yoga.com/video-classes, together with videos that support the practices in this book.

12

Breathing practices

The way we breathe can help us calm when we are anxious, energise us when we feel low in energy and balance us when we need to create some stability in our lives.

Allowing breath to move down into your belly means releasing any tension you might be holding there. A muscle held tight is not moving fully through its range of motion. There are many reasons why we might hold tension in our bellies. Surgeries and trauma to the abdomen might restrict our movement as we guard areas of the body and feel scared to move them. In addition, in the western world a flat, held-in tummy is perceived to be more fashionable and so the trend is to hold in our tummies or try to keep them flat. The reality is that our bellies should rise and fall as we breathe in and out to allow fresh nutrients to circulate through the muscles and toxic waste products to flush out. This is not happening as efficiently if we don't allow our breath to move into our abdomen.

If the abdomen is held tight and contracted, then the respiratory diaphragm may be limited in its movement, and this can prevent us breathing effectively. This can affect the pelvic diaphragm, or pelvic floor, that moves in conjunction with the respiratory diaphragm, broadening during inhalation with the movement of the respiratory diaphragm (as it draws down), and drawing in and up on exhalation. If our diaphragm is limited in its movement, then we might also need to use the secondary breathing muscles of the neck and chest to help us to get more breath into the body. This can contribute to tension in the muscles of the neck and shoulders.

When we let go of holding our belly and allow it to move outwards as we breathe in and then release when we breathe out, we give both the respiratory diaphragm and the pelvic diaphragm a chance to move. If our spine is in neutral, then it will help these important muscles be able to move and then we can literally have a sense of our whole body breathing when we inhale and exhale.

When we are breathing in fully and breathing out fully there is this internal massage in the body that is stimulating and nourishing; this is another reason why breathing is so valuable as a tool to help us to repair our body from injury and illness.

Exploring different techniques

There are many ways to breathe and, because our breathing is the quickest way to affect our nervous system, the way we breathe can change how we feel; this means different techniques can be used to energise us when we feel a bit low, to balance us when we feel distracted or to calm us when we feel anxious. When we engage in calming down, we give energy to this rather than energy to the anxiety.

The one thing that is under our control is our current thought. When we notice a thought, we have a choice. We can choose to follow that thought, ruminate, amplify or allow it to jump to another thought, and another and another. Or we can choose to observe that thought and come back to following our breath in and out. And repeat.

The *Bhagavad Gita* is an ancient Indian text or guidebook that uses the metaphor of a battlefield to symbolise the struggles we have with our mind and the desire to live our life with purpose. The text advises us to become more aware of our breath and to breathe consciously and, when our mind wanders, just to bring our attention back to our breath; in this way we will start to create a deeper sense of awareness. Chapter 5, verse 27 of the *Bhagavad Gita* says:[85]

Making outside sensations
Truly outside,
Focusing the eye
Between the eyebrows,
Making equal
The ingoing breath
And the outgoing breath
Moving in the nose.

As explained in Chapter 6, air travels into the nostrils but we also know that it alternately enters the left and right nostrils as we breathe. Every 90 minutes blood shifts from one nostril to the other so that one nostril feels more open, and one feels a bit more congested. In the yoga tradition, the right nostril being more open stimulates the left hemisphere of the brain and facilitates more rational or analytical thinking. When the left nostril is more dominant, then this stimulates the right hemisphere of the brain which is more creative and intuitive. The left nostril is associated with the moon, Chandra, and is seen to be more cooling and calming, hence breathing in through the left nostril can be a technique to calm the nervous system. Breathing in through the right nostril is associated with the sun, Surya, and is more warming and awakening and so breathing in through the right nostril is seen as being more energising and stimulating, hence this might be a breathing practice you could consider when needing more energy.

If focusing on breathing actually makes you feel more anxious, try moving with your breath. This might be opening your hands while you inhale and closing them as you exhale, or as you inhale floating your arms up towards your ears and as you exhale, lowering your arms down.

If you are new to conscious breathing, then you can explore different breathing techniques. Take time at the beginning just to notice how you are feeling in your physical, energetic and mental body, almost as if you could take a mental photograph of what it feels like to be *you* right now. Try one of the conscious breathing techniques for 5 minutes and then stop and observe what it feels like in your physical, energetic and mental body. Notice if anything changes. Do you sense any stillness? Any peace or serenity? You might be just getting a glimpse of your true nature. According to the *Yoga Sutras of Patanjali*,[86] if we can start to calm the fluctuations of our mind, we start to glimpse our true nature or true self that is inherently calm and peaceful (sutra 1.3). Chapter 6, verse 19–20 of *The Bhagavad Gita*[87] says, 'When meditation is mastered, the mind is unwavering like the flame of a lamp in a windless place. In the still mind, in the depths of meditation the Self reveals itself'.

You can try the following breathing practices seated or lying down. If you are wanting to notice if you are breathing fully and diaphragmatically then this might be easier to experience lying down (see Figure 2, page 39) or even prone on your belly (see Figure 3, page 39). If you are tired, there is more chance that you might fall asleep lying down, which might be just what you need and want. But if not, try the breathing practices sitting up, with support.

ⓒ *5 minute savasana*

The **savasana** pose gives us the opportunity to stop – to become a human being, not a human doing. It is worth taking the time to find all the props you might need to be able to lie down in relaxation. Are you warm enough? Do you need socks or a blanket to keep you warm? Our body starts to cool down when we lie down so it is worth taking the time to make sure you will be warm enough being still for five minutes. You might also want a blanket under your head or a rolled-up blanket under your knees (see Figure 15). You might prefer to bend your knees and put your feet on the floor and maybe to use a strap to hold your knees in an effortless rest pose (see Figure 16). You could play with the distance of your feet to find a place where you feel that you have space across the back of your body. Allow your physical body to settle down into the mat and feel that it is supported by the mat and the earth beneath the mat. A body scan (see next) can help to draw your attention to areas of your physical body.

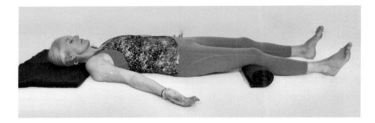

Figure 15 Savasana

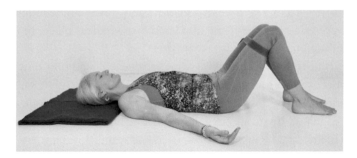

Figure 16 Savasana – bent knee version

© 5-minute body scan

A body scan is a great way to start your practice as it gives you a chance to stop and just notice what your body is telling you in this moment. Often, we have preconceived ideas about how we 'think' we feel – that we are tired, or our body is aching – but until we actually stop and observe what is really happening in the moment, we are only aware of the story we have been telling ourselves about how we 'think' we feel. We often aren't really aware of what is actually happening in this moment right now. So, by stopping we can start to get a sense of what it feels like to be us 'in this moment', and sometimes we notice things we weren't aware of – sensations in our physical body, areas that are tired or tight, but also sensations in our energetic body, areas that feel awake or full of energy or that feel a little sleepy and depleted of energy. This practice guides your attention through different areas of the body which can help it to relax. There is no need to move the areas but bring your attention to them or mentally repeat them.

You can start this practice lying down in savasana (Figure 15) with some support under your head or a rolled-up blanket under your knees. You might prefer or find it easier to sit comfortably upright in a chair with your feet on the floor. I find it easier to 'tune inwards' if I close my eyes and thereby remove the distractions that we are bombarded with every day through our eyes. You might prefer to keep your eyes open and softly gaze so that you are only really aware of the space around you and not using up lots of energy with your eyes darting around the room.

- Notice what it feels like in your physical body today.
- Feel the weight of your physical body. Does it feel relaxed or tense?
- Notice which parts of your body make contact with the chair or the floor.
- Observe your breath. Breathing in through your nose.
- Does your breath flow smoothly and evenly? Is it restricted in any way? Can you breathe down into your belly? Can you breathe into both sides of your belly or does one side receive breath more than the other side?
- Are you aware of any movement in your body just under your skin? Maybe the movements of fluid, blood and lymph, or maybe the subtle movement of energy?
- Bring your awareness down to your toes and sense them drifting away from your feet, creating space in your feet.
- Soften the soles of your feet, the front of your feet and your ankles. Feel the weight of your heels on the floor or mat.

87

- Soften your calves and feel the weight of your shins resting down onto your calves. Feel the front of your knees, the back of your knees.
- Soften your quadriceps (the muscles at the front of the thigh) and allow the weight of your thighs to release down into the mat and let your hamstrings soften.
- Soften your groin, allow all the muscles, tendons and ligaments around your hips to release and feel your legs become heavy and warm as they sink down into the mat.
- Soften your belly, lower back, middle back and upper back.
- Feel your two shoulder blades making contact with the mat. Allow them to soften down into the floor, and as they do feel your chest releasing and opening.
- Soften your biceps and triceps in your upper arm, notice the space at your elbows and forearms and the space between your forearms and your hands. Rest your awareness in the palms of your hands: are you tensing your hands or making fists? Can you soften your palms and then your thumbs, index fingers, middle fingers, ring fingers and little fingers?
- Bring your awareness to the space at the back of your neck, the front of your throat and soften the sides of your throat. Gently tilt your chin down so you feel the back of your neck and spine lengthen.
- Soften your lower jaw, gums and teeth and allow your tongue to thicken, broaden and soften. Let go of your upper jaw, gums and teeth and allow the roof of your mouth to dome upwards towards the crown of your head.
- Feel your breath caressing your nostrils.
- Allow your eyes to soften down into your head and your eyelids to become heavy. Soften the skin across your forehead.
- Feel how you are held by the mat. You don't need to do anything or hold anything; you can just let go.
- Can you allow your breath to soften with your physical body?
- Allow your mind to soften with your breath and, if you find you can't settle your mind, then invite a sense of letting go with each exhale.
- Take a few more breaths here then slowly start to bring some movement back into your physical body, preparing to come out of the body scan.

What did the body scan tell you about your body? Were you holding any tension anywhere? Were there areas of your body that were neutral and that you don't ever notice? Were you able to relax when you moved through the areas of your body? How do you feel right now?

© *5 -minute alternate nostril breathing (nadi shodana)*

Alternate nostril breathing is a wonderful breathing practice that helps to calm an overactive mind. Before you start, cross one arm over the other in a big hug and place your hands in your armpits. Breathe five breaths into your armpits (these points are said to be acupressure points that help to create a sense of emotional balance).[88] These five initial breaths may also give you a sense of being able to breathe evenly in through both nostrils. Release your hands and place them on your lap. Now you are ready to try alternate nostrils.

The following method was taught to me by Louisa McKay[89] and can be an easy way to start, especially if you are at all congested. Find a comfortable seated position on a chair or on the floor with your pelvis elevated onto yoga bricks or a bolster. Check you are sitting on your sitting bones (not rolling back onto your tailbone) and that your spine feels long.

- Gently close your fingers into the palms of your hands.
- Open up your right hand and visualise breathing in through your right nostril (see Figure 17).
- At the top of your inhale close your right hand.
- Open up your left hand and visualise breathing out through your left nostril (see Figure 18).
- Keeping your left hand open, inhale through your left nostril.
- Close your left hand, open up your right hand and breathe out through your right nostril.

This is one round. One round takes around 20 seconds. Continue for about 10 more rounds. Finish on an exhale out through your right nostril. How many rounds can you do staying focused on your breathing and the movement of your hands with your breathing?

- Finally, open up both hands, breathe in though both nostrils and exhale out through both nostrils.

Observe how you feel practising with this single focus of your breathing and the movement of your hands with your breathing. Did it help to quieten down your mind?

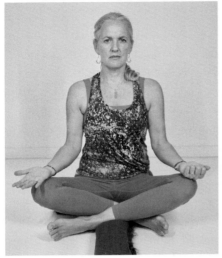

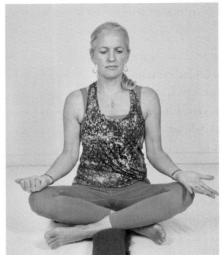

Figure 17 Alternate nostril
breathing right side

Figure 18 Alternate nostril
breathing left side

To change this practice to make it more **energising** you can try just breathing in through the right and out through the left nostrils and repeating that.

- Open your right hand and visualise breathing in through your right nostril. At the top of your inhale close your right hand.
- Open up your left hand and breathe out through your left nostril.
- Repeat in through your right and out through your left.

To change this to become more **calming** you can breathe in through the left and out through the right, and repeat.

- Open your left hand as you breathe in through your left nostril, closing your left hand at top of the inhale.
- Open your right hand as you visualise breathing out through your right nostril.
- Repeat breathing in through your left and out through your right.

© *5 minutes to calm (brahmari breathing)*

By lengthening our exhale we can stimulate the parasympathetic side of the nervous system. There are many ways to try to focus on lengthening our exhale, but one that has added benefits of sending vibrations through the body is humming. If you gently place one hand on your throat and the other hand on top and then hum, notice what you feel. Can you feel a vibration around your throat and mouth? What happens if you make different sounds? Try 'awe', then 'ooo', then 'mmm'. Does the sound lengthen your exhale? Does it also give your mind something to attend to? Did it draw your awareness inwards and away from your naturally outwardly focused attention?

When we become more aware of what is going on inside our body we build on a sense of interoception (noticing signs and signals that are going on inside of us). The more grounded and present we become in yoga, the stronger our interoceptive sense will be, which is great because our body often speaks to us through subtle sensations and we may be able to tune in to those. When we do, then we can notice if we are feeling out of ease or if the body is giving us warning signs that we might be doing too much or not taking care of ourselves. The more aware we are, the more we can tune into our body, feeding information back and being able to nurture and repair.

Humming or **brahmari** breathing (buzzing bee) is easy to do and can be incredibly uplifting as well. Lightly part your lips when you hum to explore how different sounds resonate in different areas of your mouth or throat. You might also be able to tune inwards.

- Inhale.
- Exhale and hum.
- Inhale.
- Repeat.

You can add brahmari breathing to any of the asana practices. As well as stimulating udana vayu, it will give you an anchor and help you to stay in the present moment. The longer exhale will also help you calm your nervous system and stimulate your body to rest and digest. BKS Iyengar in *Light on Yoga*[90] suggests that the humming sound in brahmari pranayama is helpful in cases of insomnia.

Ⓔ *5 minutes to energise (viloma breathing)*

Come into a comfortable seated position. Support yourself so you feel that you are sitting on your sitting bones and not rolling back onto your tailbone (see Figure 19). Starting with your arms resting on your lap and making prana mudra with your hands (see Figure 9, page 75), bring your thumb, ring finger and little finger to touch. Start to observe your breathing. Watch your breath as you breathe in and breathe out. Where do you feel pressure changes in your body when you breathe in and out? Where does your breath get stuck? Start to count your breath as you breathe in and out.

Is it easier to breathe in than breathe out? Or is it easier to breathe out than in?

Continue counting your breaths for a few rounds and see if you can start to create a sense of balance with your breath, breathing in and out to the same count.

- Take a breath in.
- Exhale.
- Breathe in halfway, pause.
- Breathe in fully and pause at the top of your inhale, lightly containing the breath and energy.
- Keep the length you have created in your spine and then exhale all the breath out fully.

Repeat.

- Breathe in a third, pause.
- Breathe in a second third, pause.
- Breathe in fully and lightly hold the breath sensing life and energy softly contained in your body.
- Keeping the length you have created in your spine, exhale all the breath out smoothly.

Repeat.

Now release the mudra and add in arm movements.

- Breathe in a third and float your arms up a third (see Figure 20).
- Breathe in a second third and float your arms up another third (see Figure 21).
- Breathe in fully and float the arms up fully (see Figure 22).
- Pause at the top. Soften your shoulders.
- Exhale all the breath out smoothly.

Repeat 2–3 more times.

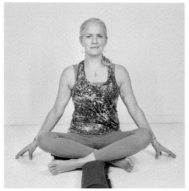

Figure 19 Seated tall

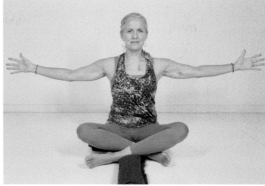

Figure 20 Viloma breathing one third

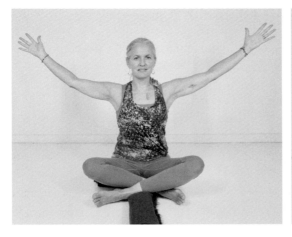

Figure 21 Viloma breathing second third

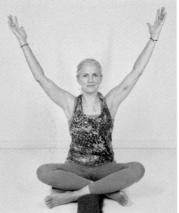

Figure 22 Viloma breathing full breath

This breathing practice is known as **viloma**. It is energising as it focuses on the inhale and drawing prana into the body. Here we are not holding the breath for long but just pausing in between breaths. Breath retentions are contraindicated for anyone with high blood pressure or a heart condition and some chemotherapy drugs can cause heart damage.[91, 92, 93] Long-held breaths can also induce anxiety and if you become short of breath it might be that you are making the pauses too long. As the quality of our breathing influences our mind, breathing should be comfortable, so if this breathing technique causes you any strain or feels restricted and increases feelings of stress and agitation, make the pauses shorter so you are not out of breath or feeling exhausted. This breathing technique should leave you feeling energised and not depleted.

Ⓒ *5 minutes to cool (sitali breathing)*

Cooling breathing techniques such as **sitali** can help you calm and take back some control, which may also help with the frequency of any hot flushes and make you feel less stressed by them. Sitali breathing is done by curling your tongue to make a straw shape that you extend out of your mouth and breathe through (see Figure 23). Having the ability to curl the tongue is genetic so if you can't do it, you can circle your mouth instead (see Figure 24) and breathe in as though you are breathing in through a straw; alternatively you could suck air in through the sides of your teeth.

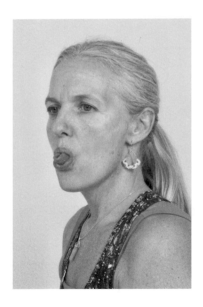
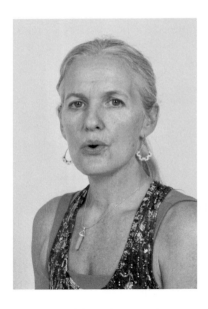

Figure 23 Sitali breathing curling tongue   Figure 24 Sitali breathing circling mouth

- Breathe in through your circled tongue or mouth and start to feel the cool air, firstly in your mouth and throat.
- Breathe out through your nose. Visualise warmth from inside your body releasing out through your nose.
- As you continue you can visualise, sense or feel the cool air travelling down into your chest and sense your chest cooling.
- Exhale, feeling warmth from inside your chest coming out with your exhale through your nose.
- Breathe in through the 'straw' or curled tongue and feel cool air travelling down into your abdomen.
- Exhale any heat/warmth out through your nose.
- Inhale sending cool breath down into your pelvis.
- Exhale, visualising or sensing any heat from your pelvis releasing out through your nose.
- Sense your whole body cooling as you breathe out.

You can stay with this breathing for a few minutes and observe any cooling sensations in your body.

We stimulate the mouth and tongue whilst breathing like this and bring a vibration or massaging effect to the vagus nerve which can help to calm the nervous system and trigger a relaxation response in the body. Deep breathing or focusing on the breath is one way we can stimulate the healthy functioning of the vagus nerve.

13

Meditation practices

All you need for meditation is a focus for your mind. This might be your breath, a word, a flower, a candle, a mantra or a phrase. It could be a physical sensation or a fixed gaze. You will also need a non-judgmental attitude about your performance. When you start to meditate you will notice that your mind is constantly wandering. You can notice where your thoughts drift off to or observe that your mind was distracted and then gently invite your attention back to your chosen focus. It is natural to wonder if we are doing it right and this is understandable, but this is also a distraction, so observe any distractions, and with a smile compassionately bring your attention back to the task of breathing or following your focus.

There are many types of meditation, and the following are a few that I use in my classes. Although the practice of meditation is challenging, it is a part of yoga that is accessible to everyone. Even at times when you are unable to move your physical body, you can use the following practices to help manage the stress and anxiety that can come with treatment for any illness. The practices can be done seated with some support for your spine (like a wall or the back of a chair) or lying down. When we become still our body temperature can drop so it might be good to have a blanket to cover yourself with whilst you meditate.

ⓒ 5 minutes' repairing light

- Lie down in savasana (see Figure 15, page 86).
- Move through the body scan (see page 87) to relax and release any tension held in your physical body.
- Bring your awareness to where your skin meets your clothing.

- Bring your awareness to where your skin meets the ground.
- Bring your awareness to where your skin meets the air.
- Sense that your body is bathed in light. All the way around your body where your skin meets your clothing, the floor and the air, there is a bright white light, a glow.
- The glow around your body can repel negativity and is protecting, nourishing and repairing.
- You can say to yourself 'I am protected by the light', 'I am nourished by the light' and 'I am repaired by the light'.
- As you breathe in, start to draw that light in through the pores of your skin.
- Sense your body filling with light – nourishing, protecting and repairing light.
- You can sense all the cells and tissues of the body being nourished by the light.
- Or you might want to send this protecting and repairing light to a certain area of your body that needs more protection, love and nurturing.
- As you breathe in, the light becomes brighter, more radiant, filling your body with vital energy.
- Feel how you are supported by the light and your body is protected by it, repelling anything negative and providing protection and nourishment. See how long you can keep that sense of a glow of light around and within your body.
- Start to bring movement back and slowly, taking time, come out of the light repairing meditation.

ⓒ ⓙ 5-minute joint space

- Lie down in savasana (see Figure 15, page 86).
- Bring some movement to your toes, wiggling them.
- Flex and point your feet.
- Invite more space down into the joint where your toes meet your feet and sense more space in your feet and ankles.
- Bend your knees and straighten your legs and bring awareness to the joint of your knees inviting more space into your knees.
- Turn your toes in andthen out, inviting more space into your hips.
- Sense the vertebrae of your spine and invite more space in-between them as you

breathe in and out. Sense your breath moving down your spine and massaging it and all the nerve endings that branch out of your spine.

• Sense your breath giving some space between your vertebrae, sensing fluidity between the joints of your spine.

• Bring your awareness to your chest and shoulders and invite more space into your shoulders. Can you breathe into the space where your arm meets your shoulder?

• Bring awareness to the space at your elbow and breathe down into that space filling your elbow with breath and sensing the fluidity of your body that nourishes your joints.

• Notice the space between your hand and forearm and breathe in and draw breath down into that space. Fill the space with breath and life.

• Bring your awareness to your hands, thumbs, index fingers, middle fingers, ring fingers and little fingers. Wiggle the fingers. Bring awareness to where the joints of your fingers meet your hands and sense space in the joints as if your fingers could drift away from your hands.

• Invite space into your neck and jaw. Relax your jaw so that your lips slightly part, and feel the space between your top and bottom jaw and allow your tongue to broaden into that space.

• As you inhale, take in light and energy with your breath and let that spacious light spread and expand throughout your body to all the joints in your body.

• Take a few moments here. When you are ready to come out roll to the side that is most comfortable to you. Press down with your top hand and come up to sit. Take a breath in and a breath out. Observe how you feel right now without judgment.

(c) 5-minute heart focus

• Start by sitting comfortably with a long spine. Sit on cushions or a support so that you are comfortable. If sitting on a chair move forward so that you are on your sitting bones and not slouching into the back of the chair.

• Bring one hand to the centre of your chest at the front and then take one hand to the back of your body so that it rests around the back of the heart. You may have one arm that is more comfortable behind your back with the palm turned out.

- Start by breathing into the hand at the front of your body and feel breath or energy moving from behind your sternum into your hand and back. Imagine that you could breathe directly into your heart and observe what this feels like. Can you sense your heart becoming fuller? More vibrant maybe? Sense it becoming full of vital energy or life force. You might even sense a colour that you feel in your heart.

- Now bring your awareness to the space behind your heart and breathe into the hand at the back of your body. This might be more challenging to feel with the eyes being at the front of the head; as a result we are front-body-focused beings, more connected to the front of our body than the back that we can't see. Can you sense your breath moving from the back of your heart to your hand? You might be aware of the beating of your physical heart or maybe the pulse of life force moving out from it. What do you associate with your heart? Is it feelings of strength and courage? Feelings of compassion and love? Can you sense these feelings radiating out into the rest of your body? Move love from your heart out to areas of your body that might need compassion or kindness right now.

Release your hands and then stay for a moment longer with the sensations that you are feeling, maybe observing how connected you feel right now or connected into this moment. How long can you keep those feelings of union as you start to move back into your day?

14

Asana practice: supine (with chair options)

(L)(E)(S) **5 minutes for digestion**

Supine crescent moon

Start supine (lying on your back). If you know that taking your arms over your head towards your ears is too challenging, then lay a bolster or blankets above your head.

Take your right foot over to the right side of your mat and then bring your left foot over to join your right. You could cross your left ankle over the right, but if that doesn't feel comfortable, keep your legs uncrossed. Both bottom cheeks should be on the mat. Then, taking your arms over your head, wiggle your head and shoulders also over to the right so that if you viewed yourself from above you would look like a crescent moon (see Figure 25).

Seated version

Sit in a chair and cross your left ankle over the right ankle. Take your right hand to the seat of the chair and stretch your left arm to the ceiling, then side-bend to the right. There is the option to bend your elbow or to take your left hand to the back of your head and point the elbow to the ceiling (see Figure 26).

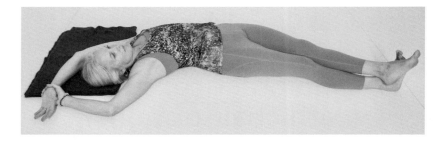

Figure 25 Supine half-moon pose

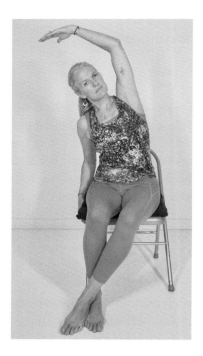

Figure 26 Seated half-moon pose

- Breathe into the left side of your body and feel that side expand. Exhale fully.
- Breathe in halfway and pause.
- Breathe in fully and pause. Feel breath and life contained in your body.

- Exhale fully, letting all your breath out.
- Breathe in a third and pause.
- Breathe in a second third and pause.
- Breathe in fully and pause. Lightly contain your breath and then exhale fully, letting all your breath out.

Repeat this sequence one more time, breathing in a third, directing breath and energy to the left side of your waist. Breathe in a third to your left rib cage. Breathe in fully to your left armpit. Exhale fully.

Continuing supine

For the supine version, if you previously crossed your ankles, uncross them and bring your feet back into the centre. Walk your arms, shoulders and head back into centre. Lower your arms and notice the difference in the left and right sides of your body.

Repeat on the other side taking your left foot over to the left side of your mat and bringing your right foot over to join your left. You could cross your right ankle over the left but if that doesn't feel comfortable, uncross your legs. Both bottom cheeks should be on the mat.

Apanasana flow

This pose stimulates apana vayu and samana vayu and is good for aiding digestion and elimination. The movements create space and then give a gentle massage as you hug your knee in.

- Interlace your fingers and, as you inhale, stretch your arms up over your head (see Figure 27).
- Exhale and hug your right knee in (see Figure 28; for the seated version, see Figure 29).
- Inhale and stretch back out, bringing your right leg back down to the floor and your arms over your head.
- Exhale and hug your left knee in.

Repeat three more times on each side.

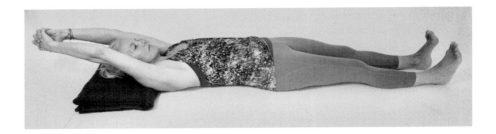

Figure 27 Full body stretch interlaced fingers

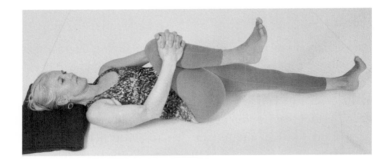

Figure 28 Hugging knees in

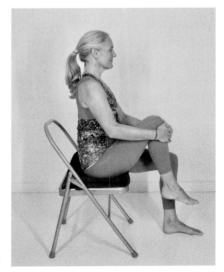

Figure 29 Hugging knees in

Next time, when you draw your right knee in, draw your left knee in as well.

- Inhale and separate your knees away from each other, keeping your feet close or touching (see Figure 30; for the seated version, see Figure 32).
- Exhale and bring your knees back to touch one another.
- Repeat 3–4 more times.
- Pause with your knees separated and breathe down into your belly. Feel your belly expand on inhale and soften on exhale. Take five breaths here.
- Exhale and bring your knees back to touching and then, keeping them together, start to circle them in one direction. If you want to stimulate your abdominal muscles, you can let go with your hands and circle your knees without the support of your hands. If that is too much, bring your hands back to your knees. Circle a few times in one direction and then change direction (see Figure 31).

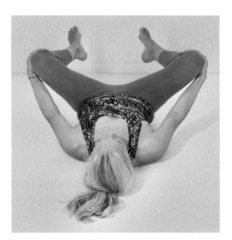

Figure 30 V-shaped bent knees

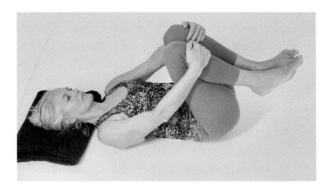

Figure 31 Circling knees

105

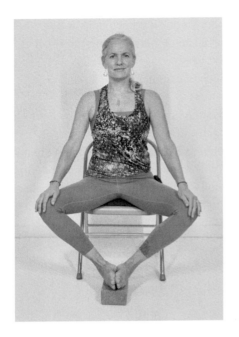

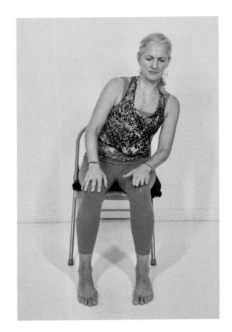

Figure 32 Seated V-shape   Figure 33 Seated circling body

Seated version

Circle your upper body, feeling your weight move from one sitting bone to the other as you move around your pelvis. Gently firm your belly to support your upper body (see Figure 33).

Release your feet back to the floor and, keeping your knees bent, widen your feet to the edges of the mat. Stretch your arms out away from your body – you can have a play with the angle of your arms and you might adjust them to get a better stretch sensation as you move into the next pose.

Twists to stimulate samana vayu

- Inhale.
- Exhale and take your knees over to the right (see Figure 34).
- Inhale and soften your chest and shoulders.

- Exhale and move your knees back through the centre and over to your other side.
- Inhale here (no movement) and soften your shoulders and arms.
- Continue moving only with your exhale, initiating the movement from your abdomen 3–4 more times.
- Then, pausing when your knees go to the right, lengthen your left knee away from your hip without straightening the leg. If you have happy knees then you could place your right foot on your left thigh and use the weight of the foot to help lengthen your left knee away from the left hip (see Figure 35).
- Take five breaths here. Exhale and change sides, repeating the hold with the knees going to the left.

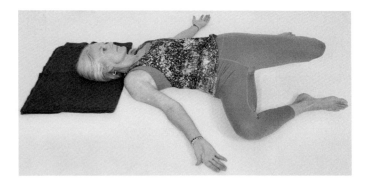

Figure 34 Wide feet twist to right

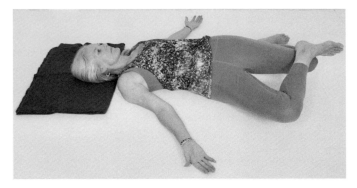

Figure 35 Wide twist with right foot on thigh

Seated version

Inhale and float your arms in line with your shoulders. Exhale and bend your elbows, turning to the left, then inhale and turn back to centre; then exhale and twist to the right.

Repeat this sequence four more times and on the fourth turn to left, stay in the twist, take your left hand to the back of the chair and your right hand to your right knee, opening your chest to the left. Take a few breaths here and then release and come back to the centre, then inhale, move your arms to be in line with your shoulders, exhale and twist to the right, taking your right hand to the back of the chair and your left hand to your left knee (see Figures 36 and 37). Finish in a seated baddha konasana (see Figure 38).

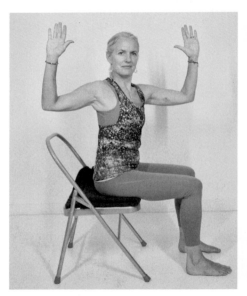 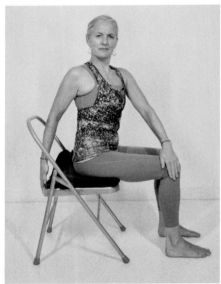

Figure 36 Seated twist goal post arms   Figure 37 Seated twist

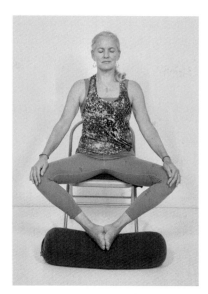

Figure 38 Seated baddha konasana

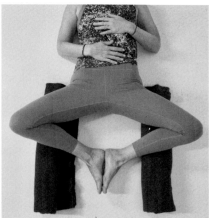

Figure 39 Supta baddha konasana

Continuing supine

To continue in the supine pose (**supta baddha konasana**):

- Bring the soles of the feet together so they touch and let the knees relax out to the sides supported by cushions or blankets (see Figure 39).
- Stay here for as long as you have time for, breathing down into your belly and feeling your belly respond to your breathing.

- When you are ready to come out use your hands to help draw your knees back up to the ceiling and then roll to the side that is most comfortable for you.
- Press down with your top hand and let your head be the last thing to come up.

Ⓢ Ⓔ Ⓙ Ⓛ 5 minutes for strength

Neck strengthening

Start by lying down on your mat with both knees bent and your feet evenly pressing down into the mat. Find the natural curves of your spine by feeling the bottom of your ribcage lightly touching and your pelvis touching the mat; you should not be actively pressing your lower back into the mat.

Press the back of your head gently into the mat so you feel the muscles at the back of your neck working. Then release and repeat 3–4 more times. This helps to strengthen the back of the neck and the muscles that get stretched when we are dropping our head forward to look at laptops or phones.

Bicycle legs

- Keeping the natural curve of your spine, inhale.
- Exhale and draw your right knee in towards you (see Figure 40).
- Inhale and extend your right leg towards the ceiling. It may not straighten and that is fine.
- Exhale and lower your right leg towards the end of your mat without changing the shape of your spine (see Figure 41). Then re-bend your right knee and bicycle your leg back towards you.
- Repeat 5–8 more times, feeling the muscles working. If you feel this in your lower back, then make the range of motion smaller so you are moving in a pain-free way.
- To finish, bend your right knee and, as you exhale, slowly lower the foot back to the floor without changing the shape of your spine.
- Repeat on the left side.

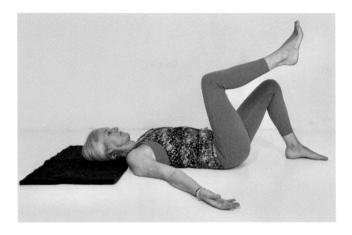

Figure 40 Bicycle legs bent knee

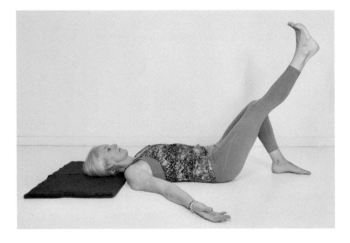

Figure 41 Bicycle legs straightening

Chair option

When sitting in a chair, exhale and draw your right knee in towards you. Then on your inhale, extend the leg away from you. Re-bend your right knee and cycle the leg back in towards you. Repeat 5–8 more times before changing sides (see Figure 29 (page 104) and Figure 42.

111

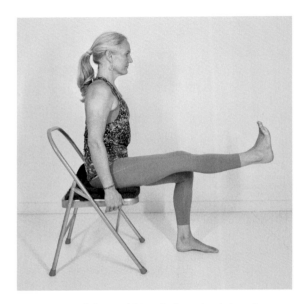

Figure 42 Seated bicycle legs straightening

Glute lifts

Your glutes are the major muscles in your buttocks.

- Lying on your back with both knees bent and feet flat on the floor or mat, lift the soles of your feet away from the floor whilst still keeping your heels in contact with the floor.
- Pressing down into your heels, inhale and lift your hips away from the floor like an elevator (see Figure 43). As you exhale, lower your hips back down.
- Repeat this nine more times. For less challenge, pause at the bottom, resting before you lift back up. For more challenge, barely touch the floor as you come down and lift straight back up.
- Lower the soles of your feet back down.

Chair option

Sitting in a chair, press your feet down into the floor or on to blocks. Can you feel the back of your legs and bottom firming as if you wanted to lift away from the chair? Repeat, firming your glutes, or, if you can, actually lift your bottom away from the chair as if you were coming up to stand. Exhale as you lower your bottom back down (see Figure 44).

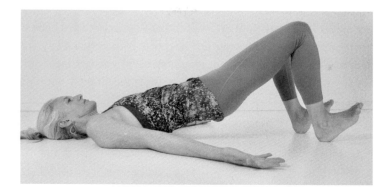

Figure 43 Bridge lifts on heels

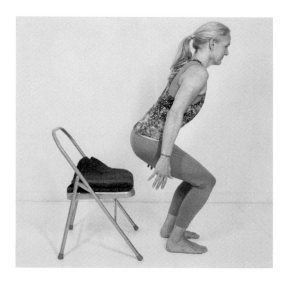

Figure 44 Sit to stand

Asymmetrical glute lifts

- Hug your right knee in towards you and feel your lower back come closer to the floor (see Figure 45).
- Lift the sole of your left foot away from the floor so you are back on your heel and then, pressing through your left heel, lift your pelvis away from the floor (see Figure 46). It may not lift very high but see if you can feel your left bottom muscles working to elevate your pelvis from the floor. Continue lifting and lowering 5–8 times. Then change sides.
- For more support place a yoga brick under your pelvis so that you have elevated the floor and your starting position is the block rather than the floor. Lift up from the block and lower back to the block instead of the floor.

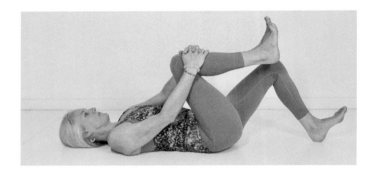

Figure 45 Preparation for asymmetrical bridge lifts

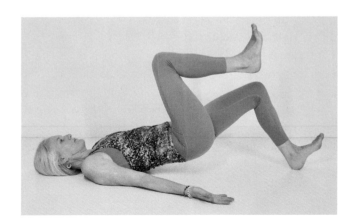

Figure 46 Asymmetrical bridge lifts on heels

Chair option

Sitting tall in a chair, extend your right leg away from you and flex the foot. Press your heel into the floor and drag it back towards the chair whilst keeping it in contact with the floor. Repeat 5–8 times, then change sides (see Figure 47).

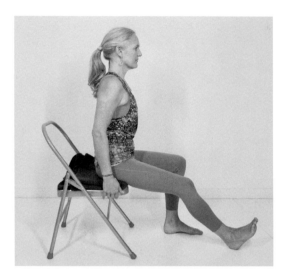

Figure 47 Seated heel drags

Clams

- Roll onto your right side. Stack your knees on top of each other and make a right angle with your thighs and pelvis and a right angle with your ankles and knees (see Figure 48).
- Slightly firm your belly so you support your lower back.
- Keeping your ankles touching, lift your top knee away from your bottom knee without moving anything else (see Figure 49). Then slowly lower your knee back down.
- Continue lifting the top knee away from the bottom knee without rocking or moving the rest of your body. Your pelvis should stay still. If you find this is challenging, then you can put your back against a wall to prevent your body moving to help the movement of the leg.

115

- Do 10 clam lifts, then roll onto your back so you can stretch out the left bottom (glute) that has been working.

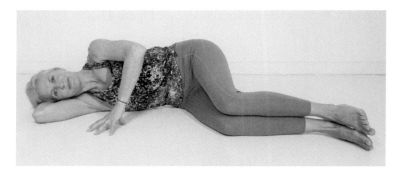

Figure 48 Side lying legs 90 degrees

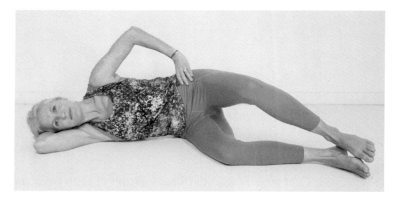

Figure 49 Clams

Chair option

Sitting in a chair, keep the big toe side of your foot (inner foot) touching the floor. Move your right knee out to the right, gently firming your outer hip/bottom area as you do, see Figure 50). Then come back to your starting position. Repeat nine more times.

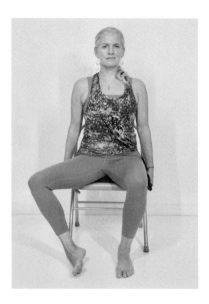

Figure 50 Seated clams

Figure-of-four stretch

- Cross your left ankle over your right thigh or bring your left heel on top of your right knee.
- Exhale, firm your belly and draw your right thigh in towards you. If you can comfortably hold on to the back of your right leg, interlace your fingers at the back of that leg (see Figure 51). If that doesn't feel comfortable then you could use the wall as a support here (see Figure 54, page 119).*

Chair option

When seated in a chair, either cross your left ankle over your right thigh or, if that is not comfortable, cross your left ankle over your right ankle. Then, fold from the top of your thighs (where they meet your pelvis) over your legs, resting your arms on your thighs (see Figure 52). Try to keep lengthening the crown of your head away from your tailbone and keeping a neutral spine.

*The wall can be a fabulous prop to help stretch out the glutes.

117

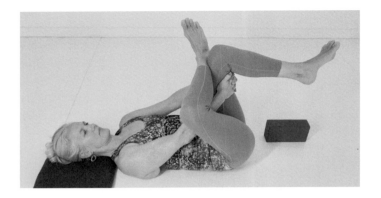

Figure 51 Figure-of-four stretch

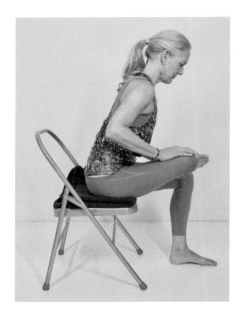

Figure 52 Seated figure-of-four stretch

Repeat clams and figure-of-four on the opposite side.

Figure-of-four with wall support

- Bring your bottom close to the wall and lean your legs up the wall, then cross your left ankle over your right thigh (see Figure 53).
- Start to bend your right knee; your foot will then slide down the wall and you should be able to press the sole of your right foot into the wall (see Figure 54). If it is too much of a stretch, either move away from the wall or slide your leg back up the wall until you find a comfortable stretch. If it is not enough of a stretch, then come closer to the wall or slide your foot down so that there is a right angle with your ankle and knee.
- Take 8 breaths here, then slide your legs back up the wall. Windscreen wiper your feet from side to side, then change sides and repeat the pose.

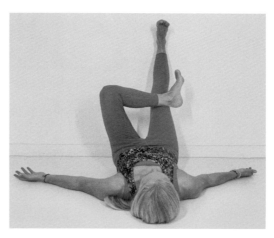

Figure 53 Preparation
for figure-of-four wall stretch

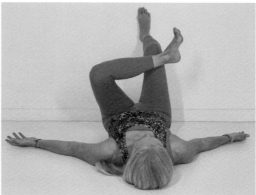

Figure 54 Figure-of-four with wall

119

Ⓛ Ⓙ Ⓒ 5 minutes to lubricate and flow

Supine downward dog/apanasana

- Lie on your back with both knees bent. Firm your belly and draw your knees in towards you (see Figure 55).

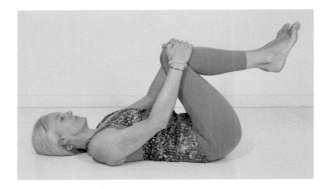

Figure 55 Hug knees in

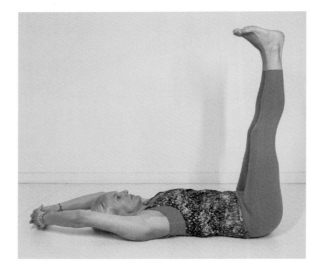

Figure 56 Supine downward dog

- Inhale and stretch your feet to the ceiling and your arms towards your ears. (There is the option to interlace your fingers to support an arm with limited range of motion – see Figure 56).
- Exhale, bend your knees and hug them back into your body.
- Repeat 5 more times. Feel the vyana energy expanding outwards into your fingers and toes.
- Release your feet back down to the floor.

Chair option

Standing, hold on to the back of a chair and walk your feet back. Keep a soft bend to your knees so that you keep a neutral spine. Breathe more into the back of your body and inflate the back of your ribcage so you lift out of your lower back (see Figure 57).

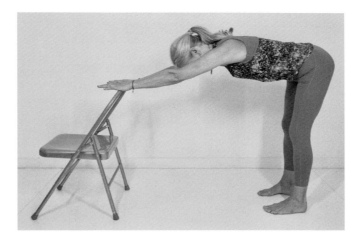

Figure 57 Downward dog with chair support

Framed baddha konasana flow

- Lie on your back with both knees bent and feet flat on the floor.
- Stretch your arms up to the ceiling and then, bending your elbows, catch hold of the opposite elbow with the opposite hand. You create a frame shape with your arms (see Figure 58).
- Inhale and stretch the frame towards your forehead or the crown of your head.

121

Open your knees away from each other. The soles of your feet may come to touch (see Figure 59).

• Exhale and firm your belly, then bring your knees towards the ceiling and elbows back towards the ceiling (coming back to your starting point).

• Repeat 5 more times.

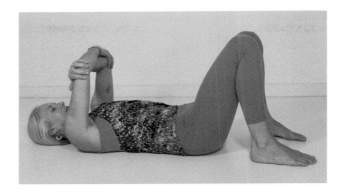

Figure 58 Frame arms and knees to ceiling

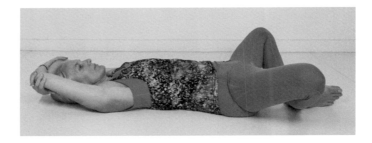

Figure 59 Frame arms and knees wide

Chair option

Sitting in a chair, inhale, stretch your arms up to the ceiling and then, bending your elbows, catch hold of the opposite elbow with the opposite hand (see Figure 58). Then stretch the frame toward the ceiling as you open your knees away from each other (see Figure 60). Exhale and bring your knees back to touch and lower your framed arms back down (see Figure 61). Repeat 5 more times.

122

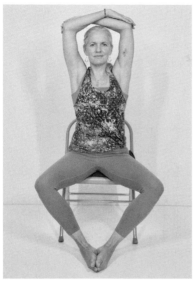
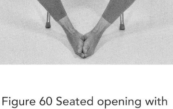
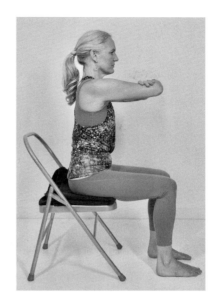

Figure 60 Seated opening with
frame arms/legs

Figure 61 Seated closing of frame
arms/legs

Framed supine twist

- Lying on your back, keep your arms in the frame position and inhale.
- Exhale and take your elbows over to the right and drop your knees to the left (see Figure 62).
- Inhale and pause in the twist.
- Exhale, firm your belly and bring your knees and elbows back to the centre; then take your elbows to the left and your knees to the right (see Figure 63).
- Inhale and pause (no movement).
- Exhale and continue taking your elbows to the opposite side to your knees, pausing on inhale.
- Continue 5 more times to each side so you finish when your knees go to the left.
- Exhale and bring your knees back to the centre and hug them into your chest.

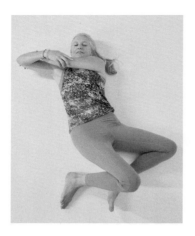
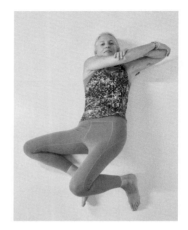

Figure 62 Twist with frame arms to right   Figure 63 Twist with frame arms to left

Chair option

Sitting in a chair, keep your feet and knees in neutral and take your framed arms to the right, opening your chest to the right (see Figure 64). Inhale, pause there and exhale, bringing your elbows back to the centre and over to the left. Inhale and pause there. Continue moving 5 more times from left to right, just moving on exhale.

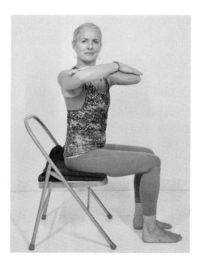

Figure 64 Seated twist with frame arms

Extend legs to the ceiling

- Lying on your back, flex and point your feet (see Figure 65).
- Circle your feet in one direction. Then change direction. This is a crucial pose for stimulating the lymphatic system and helping to pump fluid back towards the heart.

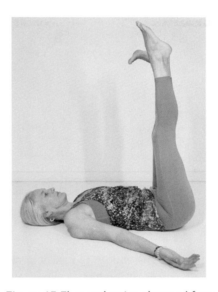

Figure 65 Flex and point elevated feet

Chair option

This does not have the same gravitational pull as the supine option but it helps to stimulate the muscles at the front and back of the lower leg which are important in that when contracting and releasing they help to pump fluid back up the legs towards the heart.

- From seated lift your heels without allowing them to splay out away from each other (see Figure 66).
- Lower your heels and then lift the balls of your feet away from the floor, keeping your heels on the floor (see Figure 67).
- Repeat, lifting your heels and then lifting everything but the heels.

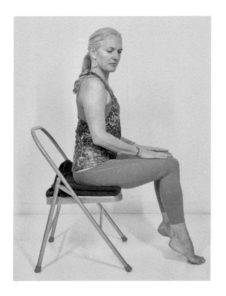

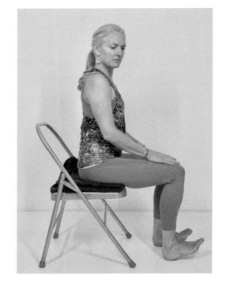

Figure 66 Seated heel raises   Figure 67 Seated sole raises

Half-wide V

Releasing tension in the inner thighs and groin can help release any restriction that may prevent the smooth movement of fluids and nerve impulses through the groin. The opening and closing also creates a pumping action to aid movement.

- Lying on your back, hug your right knee in holding onto your shin or the back of your leg.
- Extend your left leg up to the ceiling.
- Inhale and separate your two legs (see Figure 68).
- Exhale and bring your legs back together. Continue sensing that your tummy is helping to do this.
- Repeat 5 more times, then cross your left leg over your right (see Figure 69).

Place a yoga block on the floor just below your bottom.

- Inhale.
- Exhale and firm your belly and tap your right toes to the floor or the yoga block.
- Inhale and lift your toes away from the block.
- Repeat 5 times.

- Uncross your legs and extend both up towards the ceiling. Circle your ankles 5 times in one direction and then 5 times in the opposite direction. Then, keeping your right leg extended, bend your left knee into your chest and repeat the half-wide V on this side.

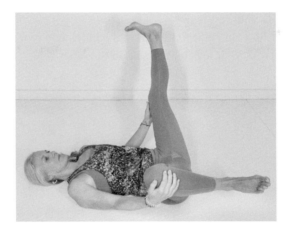

Figure 68 Release inner thigh V-shape

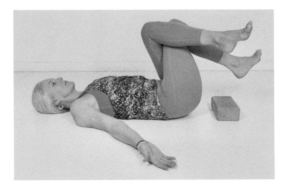

Figure 69 Crossing thighs

Chair option

- Sitting in a chair, keep your right knee bent with your right foot on the floor.
- Allow the knee to move out to the right (see Figure 70).
- Extend your left leg out to the left.

127

- Inhale.
- Exhale and bring your legs back towards each other, bending your left leg.
- Repeat 5 more times, then cross your left leg over the right.
- Position a yoga block under the toes of your right foot (see Figure 71).
- Exhale and lift your right foot (or just the toes) away from the block, flexing the foot. Relax your left leg.
- Inhale and bring your right foot back to the block and repeat 5 times.
- To finish, uncross your legs and repeat on the other side.

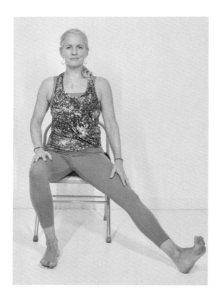

Figure 70 Seated inner thigh release V-shape

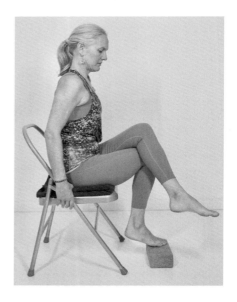

Figure 71 Seated cross thighs

You could finish this practice by elevating your legs over a chair (see Figure 72) so that your calves rest on the chair or up the wall (see Figure 150, restorative poses, page 176). With legs up the wall your bottom is very close to the wall so that your legs just sink down into your hip sockets and don't cause you any discomfort in your lower back. See Chapter 17 for more information.

Any of the 5-minute restorative practices would be a good addition to any of the asana practices and they are all done supine with the support of props.

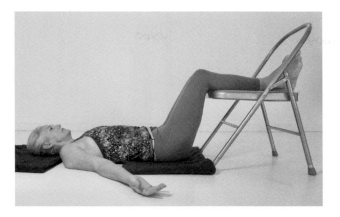

Figure 72 Legs over chair

(c)(l)(s) If you only have a minute...

... then try one pose: releasing your hamstrings with a yoga strap.
- Lie supine (on your back).
- Bend your right knee in. Take your yoga strap over the ball of your right foot and extend your leg up towards the ceiling.
- Exhale and relax your shoulders and jaw.
- Use the strap to draw your thighbone down into your pelvis, instead of pulling the leg towards your face. Keep your spine neutral. Lengthen your right hip away from your face so that you have length in the right side of your lower back.
- Keep your left knee bent or, if okay on your lower back, straighten your left leg. Flex your right foot (see Figure 73).
- Take five breaths here.
- Change sides and repeat.

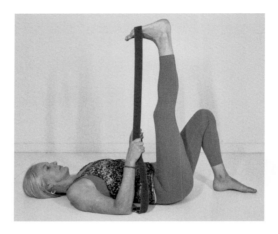

Figure 73 Supine hamstring stretch

15

Asana practice: seated

ⓙⓁⓈ 5 minutes lubricating feet and spine

Opening up the feet

Opening up the feet can help with a sense of being grounded as our feet connect us to the earth. In addition, making the feet more malleable and flexible can help with balance. So, this short sequence starts with opening up the feet which might help you to 'get back on your feet' or to feel like you can 'stand on your own two feet', which might be just what you need when you are working to repair.

This exercise can be done in a chair or elevated onto cushions or blocks on the floor. Thank you to Annie Carpenter[94] for sharing this with me.

- Take hold of your left foot and hold onto the big toe with your right hand and the second, third, fourth and fifth toes with your left hand. Start to move your hands and toes forward and back in opposition to each other so that, as you flex your big toe, you extend your other four toes. Repeat. You can move fast to warm up the connective tissue or you might move slowly (see Figure 74).
- Then take hold of your big toe and second toe (the one next to the big toe) in your right hand and the other three toes in your left hand and repeat the exercise above (see Figure 75).
- Then take hold of the big toe, second toe and third toe in your right hand and the fourth and fifth toes in your left hand and repeat the exercise (see Figure 76).
- Finally take hold of big toe, and second, third and fourth toes, in your right hand and the fifth toe in your left hand and repeat the exercise (see Figure 77).

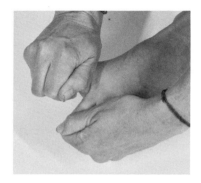

Figure 74 Opening toes: big toe vs four toes

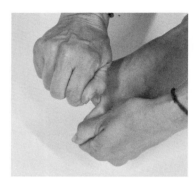

Figure 75 Opening toes: big toe and second toe vs three toes

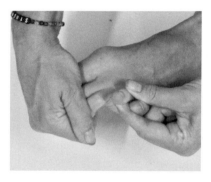

Figure 76 Opening toes: big toe, second and third toes vs two toes

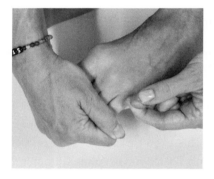

Figure 77 Opening toes: little toe vs four toes

- Then slide the fingers of your right hand in between the toes of your left foot and use your hand to help circle the toes (not the foot) in one direction 4–5 times, then change direction and circle the other way 4–5 times (see Figure 78).
- Then, fingers still in between the toes, circle the whole of your foot in one direction 4–5 times; then change direction and circle the other way 4–5 times, lubricating the ankle joint (see Figure 79).

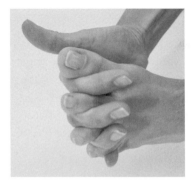

Figure 78 Circling toes

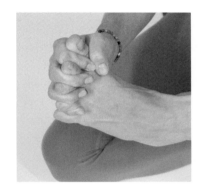

Figure 79 Circling ankle

Straighten out your legs and before you change sides notice the difference between your two feet and then repeat the exercise on the right foot.

Seaweed toes – flexing and pointing

- With your legs straight out in front of you, take your hands behind you and press down into the floor so you can feel your spine lengthen upwards. Press your hands away from your bottom so you feel the natural curves of your spine.
- Point your toes and your feet away from you (see Figure 80).
- Draw your feet back towards you, flexing your toes at the last minute (see Figure 81).
- Repeat so your feet resemble seaweed on the ocean floor moving with the current.

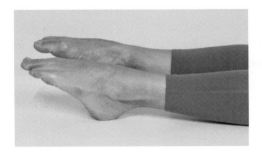

Figure 80 Seaweed feet: pointing

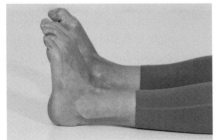

Figure 81 Seaweed feet: flexing

Cramping

It is really common to experience cramping in your feet if you are not used to moving them like this. If you do experience cramping, you can try pressing a finger above your lip and under your nose. This is an acupressure point called 'centre of the person' (GV26) and is said to relieve cramps[95] and, from experience having used this in classes, my students tell me it does actually work (see Figure 82).

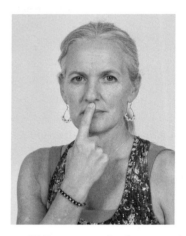

Figure 82 Pressure point for cramping

Seated cat and cow

- With your legs still straight out in front of you, take your hands behind you.
- Push your hands down into the floor to lengthen your spine and press your shoulder blades forward into your chest to help open and lift the top part of your chest by your armpits. At the same time, keep the lower part of your rib cage softening down (see Figure 83).
- Exhale and allow your chest to soften and your shoulder blades to broaden as you drop your chest in-between your arms (see Figure 84).

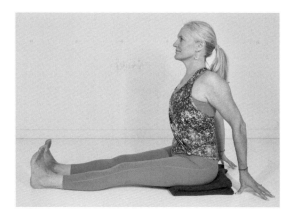

Figure 83 Seated cow pose

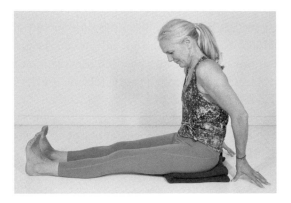

Figure 84 Seated cat pose

Sukhasana side bend

Come into a comfortable cross-legged seated position, crossing your right shin in front of the left. You can always place cushions under your thighs to give you more support or a rolled-up blanket under your ankles, as shown in Figure 85. To help keep your spine in neutral you want to sit on your sitting bones, this may mean sitting on a yoga block or folded blanket to stop you rolling back onto your tailbone. Lengthen up through your spine.

- Inhale and raise your arms out to the side and up in line with your shoulders, with palms facing forward (see Figure 85).

135

- Exhale and place your left hand on the floor. Stretch your right arm up towards the ceiling and maybe over to the left (see Figure 86).
- Inhale and move back to the centre (see Figure 85).
- Exhale and place your right hand on the floor. Stretch your left arm up towards the ceiling and maybe over to the right (see Figure 87).
- Inhale and move back to the centre (see Figure 85).
- Exhale and lower your arms.
- Repeat 2 more times.
- The third time you stretch up and over to the right, bring your right hand to the floor and bend your right elbow in towards your body so that your shoulder softens away from your ear (see Figure 88).
- Drop your right ear towards your shoulder. It won't touch your shoulder.
- Lower your left arm down until you sense a stretch or opening in the left side of your neck.
- Either hover your left hand away from the floor or rest the back of it in the small of your back. Breathe into the left side of your neck (see Figure 88).
- To come out of this position, bring your left arm over your head and, holding onto the right side of your face with your left hand, use the strength of your left arm to bring you back up to centre.

Repeat on the other side, changing the cross of your legs so that your right shin is now in front of the left.

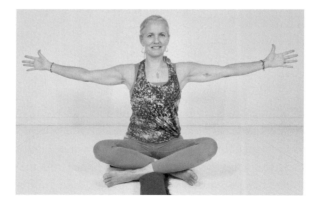

Figure 85 Arms in line with shoulders

136

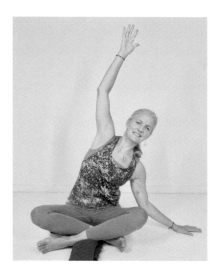

Figure 86 Side bend to left

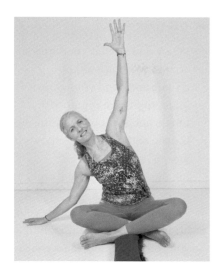

Figure 87 Side bend to right

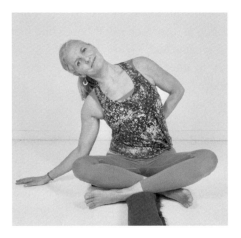

Figure 88 Neck opening

137

Goalpost twists

- Inhale and stretch your arms up, feeling like your spine grows taller with your arms (see Figure 89).
- Exhale and bend your elbows into a goalpost shape. Keeping a long spine, turn to the right (see Figure 90).
- Inhale and stretch your arms up, keeping a long spine (see Figure 89).
- Exhale and bend your elbows into a goalpost shape and, keeping a long spine, turn to the left.
- Inhale and stretch your arms up. Come back to the centre and repeat 2 more times.
- The third time you stretch your arms up, exhale and turn to the right and then bring your right hand behind you (either to the floor or to a yoga brick) and your left hand across to your right knee. If it feels more comfortable to have your hand on your left knee, keep it there. Don't use your arms to pull yourself into a deeper twist.
- Push down with your right hand to lengthen your spine. Press your right hand away from you so that your lower back feels like it moves forward rather than rounds back. Broaden across your collar bones and breathe wide into the front of your body for 5 breaths (see Figure 91).
- Inhale. Come back to the centre and exhale. Pause and notice the effects of twisting to one side.
- Inhale and stretch your arms up.
- Exhale and bend your elbows into a goalpost shape; turn to the left and pause bringing your left hand to the floor or a block behind you and your right hand across to your left knee. Try not to use your hands to pull yourself into the twist and use your breathing to deepen into the pose. Take 5 breaths on this side.
- Inhale and come back to the centre and pause. Observe what this feels like.

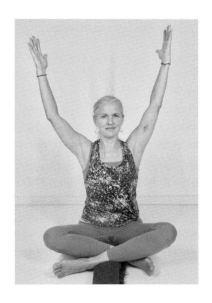

Figure 89 Lengthen arms

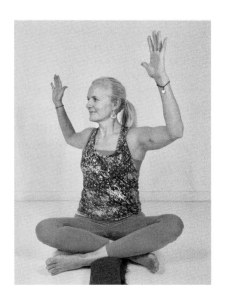

Figure 90 Goalpost twist

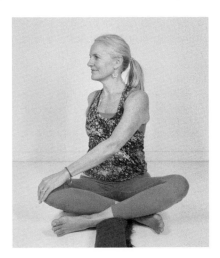

Figure 91 Seated twist

Ⓙ Ⓛ 5 minutes' opening face, jaw, neck and shoulders

Strap breathing

- Start seated on a chair or elevated on a cushion.
- Make a loop in a yoga belt and take the belt over your head and around your body, then tighten it around your lower rib cage. It shouldn't be so tight that you can't breathe in but not so loose that it will drop down when you breathe out. The belt will give you some feedback on your breathing, so start to notice the feeling of your breathing into the strap. Notice if you breathe mostly into the front of your body. (We are more aware of the front of our body because our eyes are at the front of our head.) Can you breathe into the sides of the strap? Can you feel your breath into the back of the strap? Feel your breath moving out of your front, sides and back so that you have 360 degrees of breathing (see Figure 92).

Take a breath in and yawn your mouth open as you exhale. Yawning is a great way to release your neck and throat. Then make the following small movements to open your jaw and neck. Bring your awareness to your jaw and, with your lips slightly parted, let your lower jaw move forward and back 5 times.

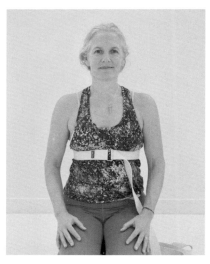

Figure 92 Strap breathing

Under jaw release

- Open your mouth so that your lower jaw relaxes and drops down. Keeping your mouth open, start to lift your chin up so you are gazing upwards (see Figure 93) and then close your mouth (see Figure 94). You should feel the stretch under your jaw at the top of your throat. Hold for 5 breaths and then release, lowering your jaw back down so your gaze is at the horizon. There is the option here to open and close your mouth while your chin is lifted as if you were biting into an apple.
- Puff out your cheeks and then move that puff of air from one cheek to the other cheek.
- Then move the puff of air around your mouth in a circular motion. Go in one direction a few times and then change direction.

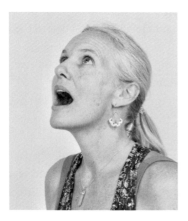 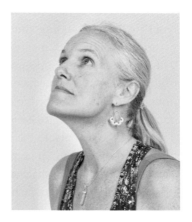

Figure 93 Open mouth, lift chin   Figure 94 Release under jaw

Face forward/face back

Can you move your face forward (see Figure 95) and then back (see Figure 96), like a chicken? This is important because we spend so much time on computers that we have a tendency to have our face forward (forward head posture) and this puts strain on the back of the neck, causing us to hunch as well as to start to lose the natural curves of our spine. Our head weighs between 4 and 6 kg but it increases in the pressure it exerts as it leans forward, and this puts a strain on the cervical vertebrae of the neck. The muscles lengthen and weaken.

When you take your face back it feels like you are going towards making a double chin, but not quite that far. It is not a tuck of the chin in towards the chest. You can also do this standing with your back to the wall and gently pressing the back of your head into the wall and then releasing or lying down as in Chapter 14, in the neck strengthening pose (see page 110).

- Without moving your face, visualise a clock and move your eyes around the clock face in a clockwise direction, from 12 back to 12. This stimulates the optic nerve and helps to calm and organise the brain.
- Without moving your face, turn your eyes to look left then turn your head to the left, feel that the movement is being initiated by the left eye (rather than your chin so it helps to keep your head in line with your spine).
- Inhale and bring your head back to the centre and then your eyes back to centre and change side.
- Turn your eyes to the right and then turn your head to the right as if the back of your right ear is guiding you into the twist. Inhale and come back to the centre with your head and eyes.
- Now experience the opposite: without moving your face, turn your eyes to the right and then turn your face to the left, keeping eyes right.
- Inhale and come back to the centre and then turn your eyes to the left and your face to the right, keeping your gaze to the left.
- Inhale and come back to the centre.
- Shrug your shoulders up to your ears so you know where you don't want your shoulders to be. Then exhale and let your shoulders just drop away from your ears.
- Make a fist with your right hand and extend your arm towards the floor. Press your fist back behind you and as you do, bring your left ear towards your left shoulder (see Figure 97). There is an option here to create a tent-like shape with your left hand and bring your fingers to the top of your head (see Figure 98).
- Press your head up into your fingers so that you feel the muscles in your neck working, then release.
- Allow the weight of your hand to help with opening the side of your neck, so now it is more of a stretch.
- Repeat the strengthening and releasing 2–3 more times. You should not pull with your hand. The hand is there to add a little bit of weight but if it feels like too much then maybe it is just that, too much. Ease out.
- Change sides, making a fist with your left hand and extending your left arm back and down as you bring your right ear towards your right shoulder. Again

there is the option to add on the tepee/tent fingers to the left side of your head and work with strengthening (pressing up) and releasing (letting the weight of your hand assist the stretch).

If you are sitting cross legged change the cross of your legs.

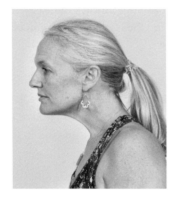

Figure 95 Face forward

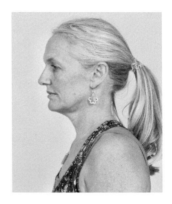

Figure 96 Face back

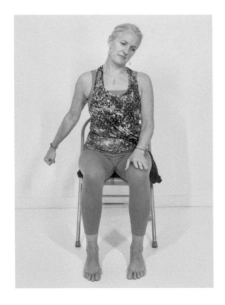

Figure 97 Neck release right side

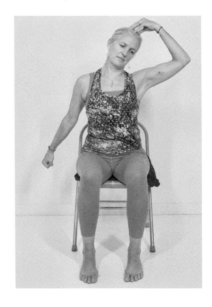

Figure 98 Lengthening neck release

143

Scarecrow arms

- Raise your arms in line with your shoulders and turn your thumbs down to the floor so the palms face the wall behind you (see Figure 99).
- Bend and straighten your elbows, keeping them in line with your shoulders, allowing your forearms to swing down and up.
- Start to swing both whole arm, still bending at your elbows but allowing your elbows to move up and down so you start to tap the backs of your hands to your lower back (see Figure 100). Repeat 5 times.
- Lower your arms down.
- Inhale and take your arms out to the sides and up in line with your shoulders. Now, keeping your palms facing upwards, tap your fingers to the back of your neck, pointing your elbows up to the ceiling (see Figure 101) and squeezing your elbows in towards your head, then re-straighten your arms out in line with your shoulders.
- Repeat 4 more times.

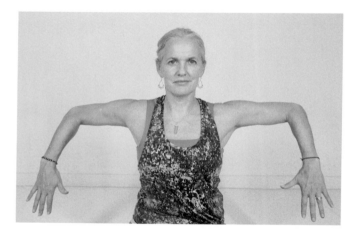

Figure 99 Scarecrow arms (internal rotation)

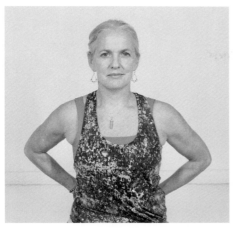
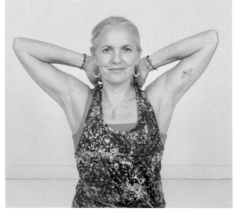

Figure 100 Tap lower back

Figure 101 External rotation of arms/hands tap neck

Cow-face (gomukasana) pose

- Tap your right fingertips to the back of your neck.
- Stretch your left arm out to the side in line with your shoulder.
- Turn your left thumb down and bend your elbow to bring the back of your hand to your lower back. Look at your left shoulder to check it isn't rolling forward. Keep the left side of your chest open. Lengthen your collar bones away from each other (see Figure 102). You can hold onto the back of your clothing to support yourself here or place a yoga strap over your shoulder so your hands can hold onto the strap with some space between them.
- Easier option: hold your top elbow with your opposite hand (see Figure 103).
- Release your arms and roll your shoulders 5 times in one direction and 5 times in the opposite direction.
- Repeat with your left elbow pointing up and your right hand to the small of your back.

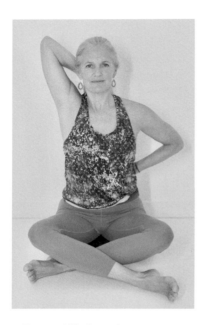

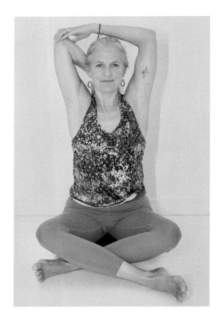

Figure 102 Gomukasana arms   Figure 103 Half-gomukasana arms

Bear-hug rib opener

- Inhale and stretch your arms out wide, away from your body.
- Exhale and cross your right arm over your left arm in a giant hug (see Figure 104).
- Inhale and stretch your arms out wide away from your body.
- Exhale and cross your left arm over your right arm in a giant hug.
- Repeat twice more on each side.
- Cross your right arm over your left and turn your elbows to the left in a small twist (see Figure 105).
- Drop your left ear towards your left shoulder and take a side bend to the left (see Figure 106).
- Inhale and breathe into your right ribcage, as if you were breathing into the spaces in-between the ribs, massaging your body from the inside out.
- Exhale and come out of the side bend.
- Inhale and bring your elbows back to the centre (coming out of the twist).
- Exhale and release your arms.

- Inhale, stretch your arms out wide and then cross your left arm over the right.
- Turn your elbows to the right.
- Drop your right ear towards your right shoulder and lean slightly to the right. Breathe into your left ribcage using your breath to create some space in the side of your body.
- Exhale and firm your belly to come out of the pose.
- Inhale and bring your elbows back to the centre.
- Exhale and release your arms.

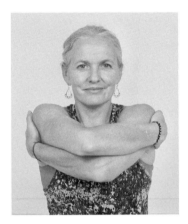

Figure 104 Giant hug right arm on top

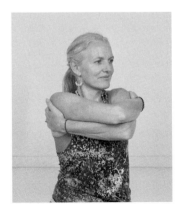

Figure 105 Cross arms: twist to left

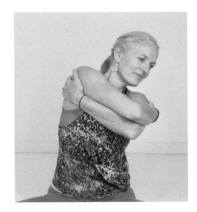

Figure 106 Cross arms: side bend to left

Shoulder circles

Bend both elbows, tap your shoulders and circle your elbows 5 times in one direction and then 5 times in the opposite direction (see Figure 107).

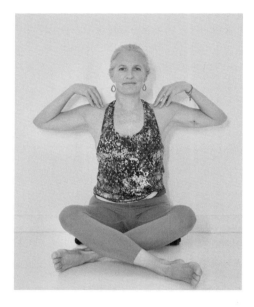

Figure 107 Circle elbows

16

Asana practice: standing

ⓈⓁⓙ 5 minutes' strengthening

Connecting to your foundations

When standing, see if you can keep a balance between your inner and outer foot. Notice if you tend to roll to one side of your foot. You might observe that there is a difference between what your right foot does and what your left foot does. If you feel your feet with your hands, rub your thumbs around the big toe mound, where the big toe joins the foot. Notice how large this surface area is. Then feel where your little toe joins your foot – your little toe mound. Then feel the large surface area of your heel. When you are standing, try to connect down through the big toe mound, the little toe mound and the centre of your heel (see Figure 108).

If you want to get a greater connection with your feet, try placing a yoga brick between your shins, as shown in Figure 109.

- Gently hug the brick so that you feel a connection to the inner part of your feet.
- Without letting the brick drop, feel as if you want to draw your legs away from the brick so you are aware of the outer edges of your feet working.
- Now see if you can get a sense of balance holding the brick whilst also slightly drawing your legs away from the brick so that you are aware of the inner edges of your feet feeling really active and balanced.
- Remove the brick and see if you can still create that same feeling of balance on the inside and outer edges of your feet.
- Try lifting one foot slowly away from the floor without changing that feeling of balance in your foot. Then change and lift the opposite foot without changing anything about your foot.

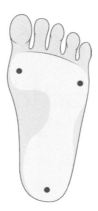

Figure 108
Points of contact
for foot

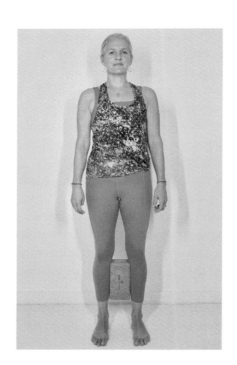

Figure 109
Block support in
tadasana

Calf release

- Tightly roll up half of your mat.
- Step the ball of your left foot onto the roll and step your right foot over the roll onto the floor in front (see Figure 110).
- Feel the ball of your left foot pressing into the roll and notice if you are shifting on to the little toe on the side of your foot. Can you bring more weight into the big toe joint, so that you are broad across the ball of your foot?
- If you want more stretch, slide your right foot a little further away from the left foot.
- If balance is challenging, stand close to a chair or wall for support.
- Try to add on a little bend to the left knee. Keep the ball of your left foot broad.

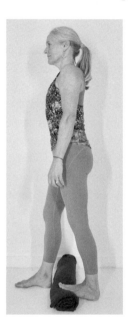

Figure 110 Calf release
with rolled blanket

- Whilst continuing to stand on the roll with your left foot, take one breath in. Take one breath out.
- Breathe in, counting 3, 2, 1.
- Breathe out, counting 4, 3, 2, 1.
- Breathe in, counting 4, 3, 2, 1.

- Breathe out, counting 5, 4, 3, 2, 1.
- Breathe in, counting 5, 4, 3, 2, 1.
- Breathe out, counting 6, 5, 4, 3, 2, 1.
- Continue with this counting routine unless it feels like it strains your breathing. If it does, then find a count that works for you.

Then step off the roll. Stand so that your feet are spaced so that they fully support you and observe your two feet. Notice if one feels more grounded or connected to the floor.

Repeat the exercise with the ball of your right foot on the roll and your left foot in front.

Dynamic calf strengthening

- Stand with your feet spaced so that you feel you are supported and stable.
- Hold your yoga strap at hip level about shoulder distance apart and then pull out on the strap (see Figure 111).
- Inhale and slowly lift your heels without them splaying out away from each other (see Figure 112), lifting your arms at the same time.
- Exhale and lower your heels and arms back down.
- Now try slowing down the movement so that it fits your breathing.
- Breathe in as you lift arms and heels and count 5, 4, 3, 2, 1.
- Breathe out as you lower your heels and count 5, 4, 3, 2, 1.

Repeat one more time, moving with your breath.

Chair option

- Staying seated, inhale, lift your heels and pull out on your yoga strap.
- Float your arms up.
- Exhale and lower your heels as you float your arms down (see Figure 113).

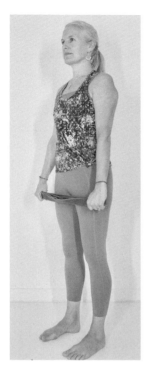
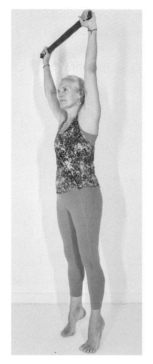
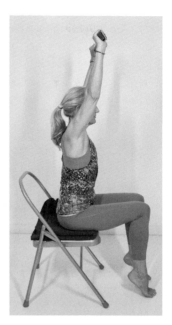

Figure 111 Shoulder distance strap

Figure 112 Calf and arm raises

Figure 113 Seated calf and arm raises

Dynamic chair

- Standing, take the strap behind you at hip level and hold it about shoulder distance apart.
- Inhale and pull out on the strap to straighten your arms, moving away from your body in a pain-free way (see Figure 114).
- Exhale and bend your knees. Sit back into chair pose (see Figure 115).
- Inhale and straighten your legs.
- Exhale and lower your arms back down towards your bottom.
- Inhale and pull out on the strap, counting 5, 4, 3, 2, 1.
- Exhale and bend your knees, sitting back into an imaginary chair, counting 5, 4, 3, 2, 1.

153

- Inhale and straighten your legs, counting 5, 4, 3, 2, 1.
- Exhale and lower your arms, counting 5, 4, 3, 2, 1.
- Repeat one more time, moving with your breathing. There is the option to add on humming (see page 91) with your exhale.

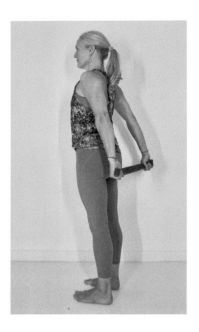 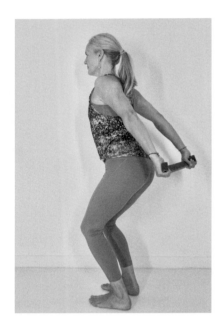

Figure 114 Chest opening with strap   Figure 115 Chair pose with chest opening

Chair option

- Starting seated, as you inhale press through your feet to lift your bottom away from the chair and, on your exhale, lower yourself back down to the chair.
- You can hold on to the back of the chair and lift your chest to your chin as if you are inflating your chest by breathing into it to open up the front of your body; keep your front ribcage drawing into your body (see Figure 116).

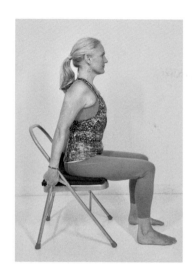

Figure 116 Seated chest opening

Warrior I

Starting with your feet hip-distance apart, step your left foot back to the left side of your mat so that you feel balanced and stable. Stay on the ball of your back (left) foot. This makes balancing more challenging so you might like to be close to a wall.

- Interlace your fingers and place them on top of your head (see Figure 117).
- Inhale and lengthen your head up into your hands (without lifting your chin) so you feel that your spine is long and neutral.
- Exhale and point your left elbow up and your right elbow down and to the right so you create space on the left side (see Figure 118).
- Inhale and come back to neutral.
- Exhale and open your chest to the right, pointing your right elbow back and your left elbow forward so you come into a twist (see Figure 119).
- Inhale and come back to the centre and neutral.
- Repeat 4 more times.

If you want to rest in between each of these moves you can straighten your legs when you come back to centre, release your arms for a few breaths and then repeat.

Then change sides, stepping your right foot back, and repeat the sequence.

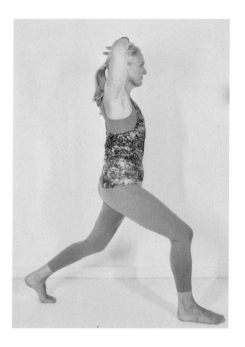
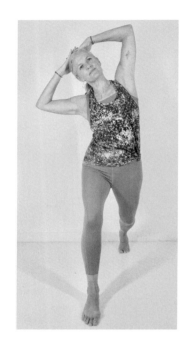

Figure 117 Warrior I with hands on head   Figure 118 Warrior I with side bend

Chair option

•   Repeat the above instructions using a chair for support under your right thigh, as shown in Figure 120.

Then stand for a moment (or sit if you've gone for the chair option). Place one hand on your heart and the other on your tummy. Breathe in fully. Breathe out fully. (See Figure 121.)

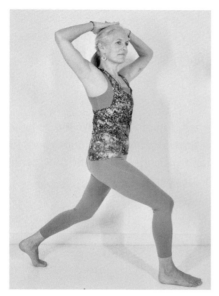

Figure 119 Warrior I with twist

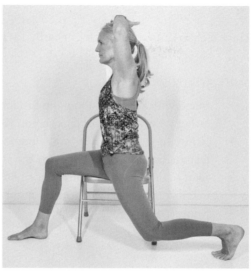

Figure 120 Warrior I with chair support

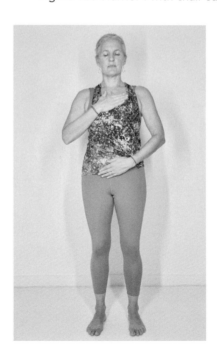

Figure 121 Checking back in
with breath

157

Ⓢ Ⓛ Ⓙ 5 minutes' hip opening

Have a chair or two yoga bricks nearby for the final poses.

Gate opening

- Stand with your feet about hip distance apart. Imagine you have the yoga brick in-between your lower legs so you feel a sense of balance through your feet.
- Bring your weight into your left foot and pick up your right foot, without leaning backwards or changing the shape of your spine.
- Start to draw a circle with your right knee (see Figure 122).
- Circle 5 times in one direction and then the other.
- Repeat, lifting your left knee.

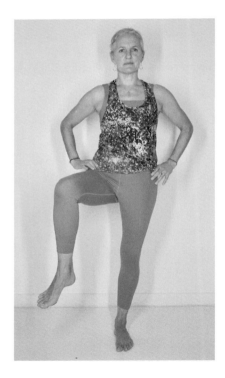

Figure 122 Circling knee

Dynamic Warrior II – side-angle pose

- Step your feet wide apart and face the long edge of your mat. Check your feet are in line with each other.
- Turn your right toes out 90° and pick up your left heel and turn it slightly out (see Figure 123).
- Press down through both feet and feel that there is even weight in both. Keep that as you start to bend your right knee so that your right knee is working towards being in line with your right ankle.
- Press down evenly through both feet.
- Check your front knee isn't rolling in towards your big toe. If you think it is, you can lift your right heel and then stretch out from your inner thigh to your inner knee and guide your knee towards your middle toes. Then lower your right heel down and press out through your inner and outer foot.
- Inhale and raise your arms out to the side in line with your shoulders or maybe even higher than shoulder height (see Figure 124).
- Exhale and draw your right thigh back into your pelvis and windmill your right arm across your body and your left arm over your head as you lean to the right. Come into a modified version of the side-angle pose (see Figure 125).
- Inhale and come back into Warrior II (see Figure 124).
- Exhale, then straighten your right leg and lower your arms down (see Figure 123).
- Repeat 3–4 more times, moving with your breathing. There is the option to add on humming with your exhale.
- Then, next time you come into the modified side-angle pose you can bring either your right hand or your right forearm to your right thigh.
- Then make circles with your left elbow (see Figure 126).
- Gravity wants to pull you towards the floor so drawing your pubic bone towards your belly button helps to incorporate your tummy muscles to turn your belly button and rib cage towards the ceiling and open your chest towards the ceiling. Check that you haven't gone into a back bend and that your chest is opening but your ribs aren't poking out. Breathe into the back of your body.
- You might start to unfurl your left arm and make circles with it. After a few circles, change direction.
- To come out of the pose, press down into your feet and use the strength of your legs to come up to stand.

- Turn your right toes in and your left toes out 90° to repeat on the other side.

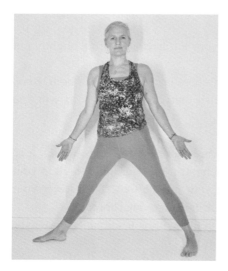

Figure 123 Feet wide arms by side

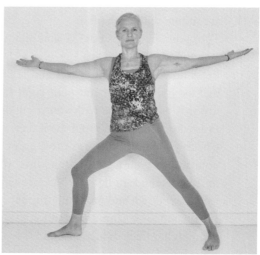

Figure 124 Warrior II

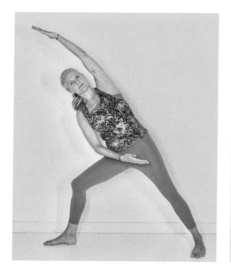

Figure 125 Preparation for
side-angled pose

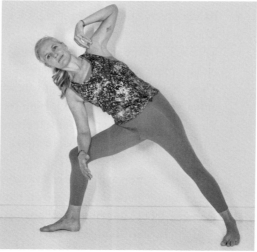

Figure 126 Side-angled pose

Chair option

Figure 127 shows how to practise Warrior II and the side-angle pose from a seated position.

To create more challenge with the chair:

- Place the chair against a wall so that it can't slide.
- Place your right foot on the chair and step your left leg back (see Figure 128).
- Turn your right toes out to the right.
- Slide your left heel slightly out.
- Inhale and raise your arms out to your side in line with your shoulders or maybe even higher than shoulder height (see Figure 129).
- Exhale, draw your right thigh back into your pelvis and windmill your right arm across your body and your left arm over your head as you lean to the right. Come into a modified version of the side-angle pose (see Figure 130).
- Inhale and come back into Warrior II.
- Exhale, straighten your right leg and lower your arms down.
- Repeat 3–4 more times, moving with your breathing.
- Then, next time you come into the modified side-angle pose you can bring either your right hand or your right forearm to your right thigh.
- Then make circles with your left elbow.
- Gravity wants to pull you towards the floor so draw your pubic bone towards your belly button to help your tummy muscles turn your belly button and rib cage towards the ceiling and open your chest towards the ceiling. Check that you haven't gone into a back bend and that your chest is opening but your ribs aren't poking out. Breathe into the back of your body.
- You might start to unfurl your left arm and make circles with it.
- After a few circles change direction and repeat.
- To come out of the pose, press down into your feet and away from each other to come up to stand.
- Step off the chair and repeat on the left side.

If balance is challenging, then you can have a wall behind you and stand close to it for support.

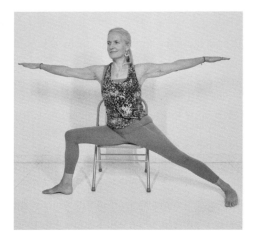

Figure 127 Warrior II with chair support

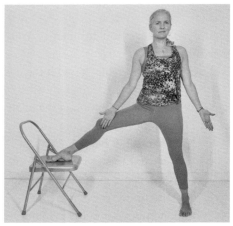

Figure 128 Feet wide with chair

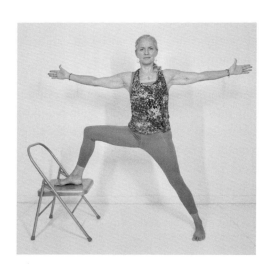

Figure 129 Warrior II with chair

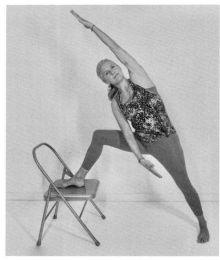

Figure 130 Side-angled pose with chair

Horse stance to tree

- Step your feet wide apart, turn your toes out and bend your knees; this is called horse stance. Check to see if your knees are going in the same direction as your toes and, if not, adjust your feet so your knees and toes are going in the same direction.
- This can be made easier by having your feet closer together or more challenging by having them wider apart.
- Bend your knees, elevate your arms and take them into a diamond shape (see Figure 131).
- Inhale here.
- Exhale and push off with your left foot so that you bring your weight into your right foot and step your left foot to join the right, or even bring your left foot to your right leg so you balance for a moment in tree pose. Your hands can come into a prayer position or to your hips for more support (see Figure 132).
- Inhale and step back into horse stance (see Figure 131).
- Exhale and push off with your right foot so that you bring your weight into your left foot and step your right foot to join the left or even bring your right foot to your left leg, so you balance for a moment in tree pose. Your hands can come into a prayer pose or to your hips for more support (see Figure 133).

Repeat 4 more times to each side, maybe staying for a few breaths in tree pose. If staying in the pose, hug the outer hip of the standing leg in; it should feel like your leg and foot press evenly against each other, so you don't collapse into your outer hip.

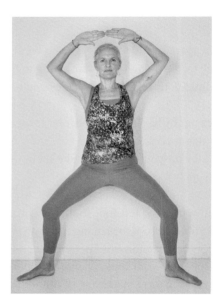

Figure 131 Horse stance with diamond arms

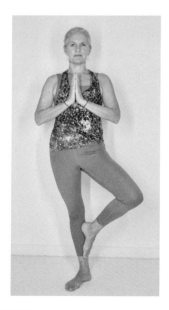

Figure 132 Tree pose: balance on right

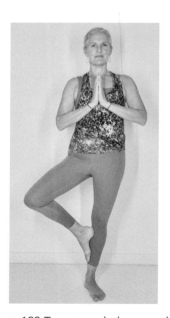

Figure 133 Tree pose: balance on left

Horse stance to forward-fold

From horse stance, with knees bent, bring your hands to your thighs. Press down onto your thighs so you feel your spine is long and neutral. Then folding at the top of your thighs, fold forward keeping your spine long (see Figure 134).

- Without changing the shape of your spine see if you can bring your hands to a chair or to blocks (see Figure 135).
- Turn your toes so they point forward, and your feet are parallel to the short edge of the mat.
- Press down into the balls of your feet and start to lift your sitting bones up; this will start to straighten your legs but resist the temptation to press your knees back to straighten your legs.
- Keep the shape of your spine so you don't feel you are rounding. If you do feel your spine rounding, then bend your knees but keep pressing down with the balls of your feet and lift your bottom away from your feet.
- Take 5–8 breaths here.
- To come out, move your heels in, then your toes in, and heel-toe your feet until they come in closer, about hip distance.
- Bend your knees, as if you are sitting into an imaginary chair, sweep your arms forward and up (see Figure 136), keep your spine long and come up to stand using the strength of your legs (as opposed to rounding your spine).

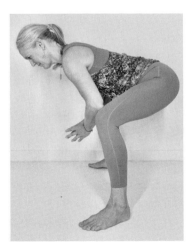

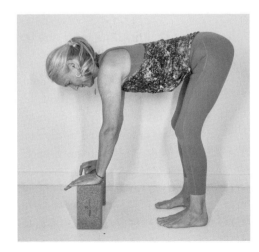

Figure 134 Forward fold in horse stance   Figure 135 Forward fold with brick support

165

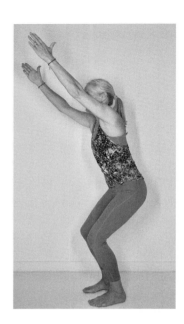

Figure 136 Chair pose

ⓈⓁⒿ **5 minutes to balance**

Have a chair nearby.

Standing neck, shoulder and chest release

- Standing, turn your palms forward.
- Inhale and raise your right arm out to the side of your body and up towards your ear. Turn your gaze to the right so you are looking at your arm (see Figure 137).
- Exhale and bend your right elbow out to the right and slightly back so you feel your chest opening and turn your gaze to the left (see Figure 138).
- Inhale and bring your gaze back through the centre and to the right as you straighten your arm back up towards ceiling.
- Exhale and bend your right elbow out to the right as you gaze to the left.
- Repeat on the right side 3 more times. Then lower your arms.
- Then close your eyes and notice the height of your two shoulders. Notice if your arms are the same length and if you are aware of any sensations in your chest and arms.

Repeat with your left arm, turning your gaze to the right as you bend your left elbow.

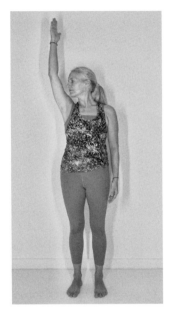

Figure 137 Right arm raise, gaze right

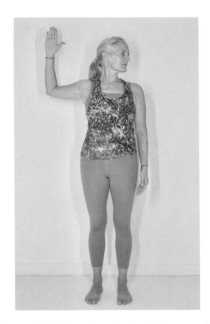

Figure 138 Elbow bends to right, gaze left

Marching

- Take one hand to your lower ribs and one hand to your lower belly.
- Exhale and gently sense your two hands drawing towards each other and a sense of your core engaging (see Figure 139). This is very subtle. If you go too far you will feel your spine rounding. Take a mental snapshot of what it feels like here with your spine in neutral and your core engaged.
- Sense both feet on the mat and feel your big toe mound, little toe mound and the centre of your heel grounding down into the mat.
- Inhale and stretch your arms forward and up (see Figure 140).
- Exhale, lower your arms down and lift up your left knee (see Figure 141).
- Inhale and stretch your arms forward and up as you lower your left foot.
- Exhale, lower your arms and lift up your right knee.
- Inhale and repeat 2 more times on each side.

Incorporating our core when we are moving and lifting our knees means less strain on our knees. Try this when climbing stairs.

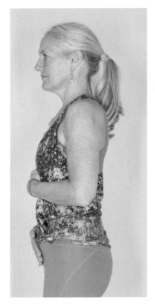 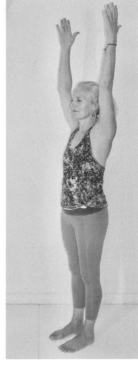 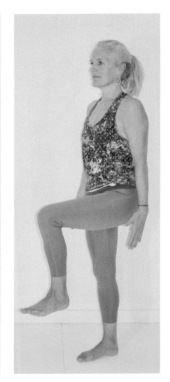

Figure 139 Drawing ribs to pubic bone core support | Figure 140 Inhale stretch tall | Figure 141 Marching raise left knee

Chair option

For more support, start with your left foot on a chair.

Inhale and float your arms up.

- Exhale and lift your left heel (see Figure 142). You can also lower your arms or place a hand on the wall for more support here.
- Continue with the option to work on lifting your whole foot on exhale once you gain more strength.

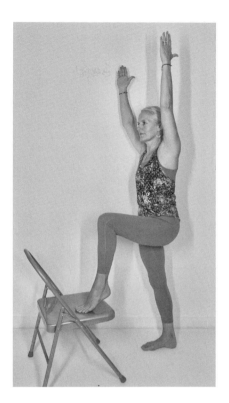

Figure 142 Marching raise with chair support

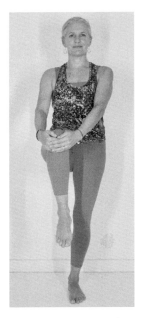

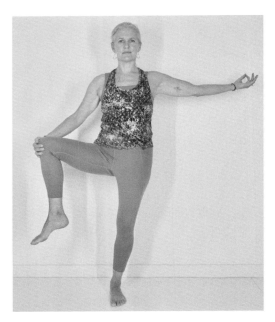

Figure 143 Gently hug knee

Figure 144 Knee to right, arm to left

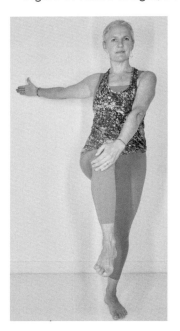

Figure 145 Balance twist

March open and close

- Inhale and lift your arms up (see Figure 140).
- Exhale, firm your belly and lift your right knee.
- Gently hold your knee with both hands (see Figure 143).
- Inhale and take your knee out to the right with your right hand, taking your left hand out to the left (see Figure 144).
- Bring your knee back to the centre.
- Exhale and take your knee to the left with your left hand, taking your right hand out to the right (see Figure 145).
- Inhale and bring your knee back to the centre.
- Exhale and lower your foot back to the mat.

Trikonasana

- Step your feet wide and face the long edge of your mat. Check your heels are in line with each other, or your front heel is in line with the arch of your back foot. Turn your right toes out 90 degrees and pick up your left heel and turn it slightly out (see Figure 123, page 160).
- Press down through both feet and feel that there is even weight in both. Check if your spine is in neutral. If you aren't sure, you can repeat the first stage of marching (see page 168), to sense a firming of the front of your body.
- Bring your hands to your hips and explore the side-to-side movement of your hips. As you exhale, shift your hips to the left and feel how you tip laterally to the right (see Figure 146). Press down with your feet and, using the strength of your legs, inhale and come back to neutral.
- Lengthen your arms out in line with your shoulders. Reach out through your right hand as your pelvis shifts to the left. Your right hand can come down to a chair (see Figure 147). Or you might bring your hand to your leg or a block.
- Then turn your left palm back so it faces away from your body. Bend your elbow and take the hand to the back of your pelvis or maybe wrap it round towards your right thigh. Press the back of your hand into your tailbone to encourage your tailbone to draw in towards your body. (You might also experience this as your pubic bone drawing towards your face).
- Look at your left shoulder. See if you can roll your left shoulder to the ceiling so that the left side of your chest broadens and opens.
- Breathe into the back of your ribcage so the back of your body broadens, and

171

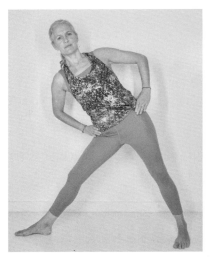 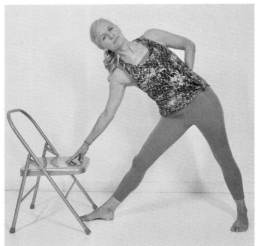

Figure 146 Preparing for trikonasana

Figure 147 Trikonasana with chair support

your ribs at the front don't poke out into your clothing. Then stretch the top (left) arm to the ceiling.

- Press down evenly with both feet and allow your right sitting bone to drop down and back towards your left foot so your pelvis shifts to the left.
- Take a few breaths here.
- Finish with your left hand on your hip ready for the half-moon pose.

Transitioning to half-moon pose

- Put a bend in your right knee. Step your left foot in a little closer so that you start to put weight into your right foot preparing your body to balance (see Figure 148).
- Keeping your hand on the chair for more support, start to lift your left foot away from the floor so you are balancing on your right leg (see Figure 149).
- Press the top of your right thigh back. This may initially bring weight into your heel so then redistribute the weight in your foot so that you feel the weight is in the ball of your foot as well.

172

- Check you are not locking out your leg. Aim for a micro-bend in your leg so that the balancing leg looks straight but you know it isn't fully straight.
- Keep the left side of your chest open.
- Bring your front ribs towards your hip bones; you might 'feel' your core working. Then lengthen out through your sternum (breast bone) so you feel

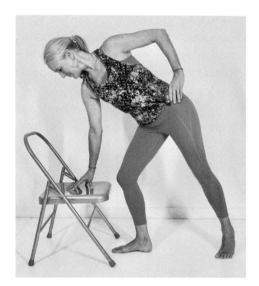

Figure 148 Preparing to balance

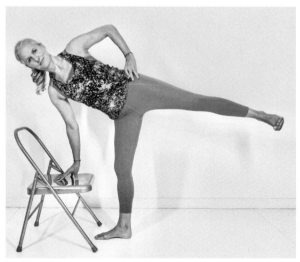

Figure 149 Half-moon pose
with chair support

long in your spine and not rounding or arching.

- You can keep your left hand on your hip, or you can stretch the top (left) arm up towards the ceiling. Take a few breaths here.
- To come out, bend your standing leg. Reach back with your lifted leg and bring it back to the mat so you come back into trikonasana.
- Press down through your feet and use the strength of your legs to come up to stand.
- Step your feet back together. You can do this by heel-toeing your feet in towards each other or soften your knees and hop your feet back together.
- Repeat trikonasana and the half-moon pose on the left side.

Finish by taking a few breaths with one hand on your heart and the other on your belly. Observe how you feel right now without judgment.

17

Restorative practices

Restorative practices give you a chance to slow down, find some stillness, some space in your body, and to be held and supported in a comfortable shape that should feel totally delicious to be in. That sounds great on paper but if, like me, you have been brought up with a 'more is more' attitude, then practising 'less is more' can feel really difficult. Suspending thoughts, judgments and ideas and 'doing' nothing but just 'being' can make you hugely aware of how busy your mind is and how hard it is to do 'nothing'. But if you do find five minutes to take a supported restorative pose you might observe how it helps to release tension and open your body, creating a sense of balance in the body. The benefits of restorative yoga include supporting the immune system function, promoting the relaxation response, calming the nervous system to shift into 'rest and digest' (see page 39) and helping with sleep.

(E)(L)(C) 5 minutes to energise

Viparita karani with blankets

This pose is calming for the nervous system, and it turns your body upside down thereby giving it a break from its normal functioning of having to pump blood back towards the heart. This can leave you feeling more energised than when you started, and therefore it is calming *and* energising. It can help to encourage movement of fluids back down your legs, relieving any swelling of feet and ankles so is great for the lymphatic system.

- Place two folded blankets near a wall.
- Sit with your right outer hip on the blanket so your sit bones are close to the wall.

175

- Use your hands behind you on the floor to support you as you roll your sacrum onto the blankets and your legs up the wall. Push your hands into the floor to push your hips closer to the wall.
- Gently lower your head and shoulders to the floor, keeping your hips close to the wall so that your legs don't lean but are supported and you feel your thighbones descending down into your pelvis (see Figure 150). Stay for 5 minutes.

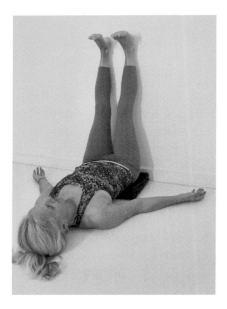

Figure 150 Legs up the wall

Legs over a chair

An alternative to this is legs over a chair. You need to have two folded blankets, one for underneath your head and one that will go under your pelvis and lower back to keep your pelvis in neutral. Place a chair in front of you and sit on a folded blanket facing the chair. Take your legs over the chair so that your calves rest on the chair seat, lower yourself onto the mat (see Figure 72, page 129).

Adjust the blankets if needed so that your head is supported and there is space at your neck and your pelvis is in neutral.

Breathe down into your belly. Can you sense your belly rising as you breathe in and falling as you breathe out? Can you sense the internal movement of your body when you breathe? Breathing fully and diaphragmatically massages your lymphatic duct, the largest lymph duct in the body, and encourages the movement of the fluid back up to the heart.

Visualise fluid containing infection-fighting white blood cells passing through your lymph nodes, filtering out bacteria, waste and toxins. Then your filtered lymph fluid flowing back into your bloodstream and being carried towards your liver and kidneys and bladder ready for elimination.

- Inhale.
- Exhale and count 3, 2, 1.
- Inhale and count 3, 2, 1.
- Exhale and count 4, 3, 2, 1.
- Inhale and count 4, 3, 2, 1.
- Exhale and hum for 4, 3, 2, 1 counts.
- Inhale and count 4, 3, 2, 1.
- Exhale and hum for 4, 3, 2, 1 counts.

Continue for three more rounds. You might increase the inhale and humming exhale to a count of 5 if that feels comfortable.

Adding 'the bee'

You could add **brahmari** mudra (the bee). Bring the index finger of each hand to the base of the thumb and the tip of your thumb to the inside of your middle finger, close to the fingernail. This mudra is said to help strengthen the immune system (see Figure 151).

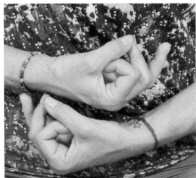

Figure 151 Brahmari mudra

ⓒ Ⓛ 5 minutes to create maximum space

Supported supta baddha konasana

This pose can help to lift the diaphragm off the stomach and liver and can relieve indigestion, flatulence and/or diarrhoea. When the diaphragm moves it massages the thoracic duct (the main duct in the lymphatic system) so can also be really supportive for the lymphatic system.

- If you have a yoga belt, long belt or long scarf, create a large loop in it.
- Place a bolster, or pile of folded blankets, vertically a few inches behind you and sit in front of it with your knees bent.
- Place a folded blanket on the other end of the bolster for your head.
- Bend your knees to opposite sides and bring the soles of your feet together.
- Bring the belt over your head and around your sacrum/pelvis.
- Pull the loop in front of you over your toes and underneath your feet so that the sides of the belt are on the inside edges of your legs.
- Now bring your feet closer to your pelvis and tighten the belt so that it is holding your legs close to your torso (see Figure 152). Don't make the belt so tight that you feel a pull on your knees.
- Lie back over the bolster and place your head on the blanket so that your chin doesn't tilt back.
- With your hands, slide your sacrum and buttocks towards your feet so that your lower back feels long. If you feel any compression in your lower back, you may need to slide a bit more off the bolster towards your feet.
- Pull your shoulder blades away from your neck and roll the outer edges of your shoulders down so that your chest spreads from the centre to the sides. Let your arms release to your sides on the floor, spreading away from your chest, rotated outward, palms facing up.
- Place a cushion or yoga block underneath the outer edge of each leg. Close your eyes and rest for as long as you want to, up to 10 minutes. Sense your breath moving down into your belly and allow your shoulder blades to feel as though they are sliding down the sides of the bolster and allowing gravity to open up your chest.
- Bring your awareness into your abdomen and breathe fully into your belly, allowing it to rise on inhale and fall on exhale.

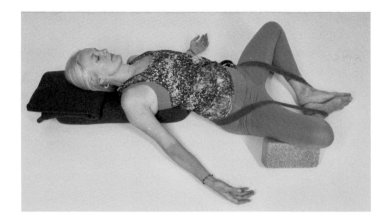

Figure 152 Supta baddha konasana restorative

Ⓒ Ⓛ 5 minutes to release tension in the front body

Supported bridge

This can be a really great way to open the front of the body, chest, belly and hips and to release tight hip flexors whilst still being restorative and promoting repair. As the legs are higher than the heart it aids the movement of fluid back towards the heart.

This pose can be done in a few ways, so here are two possibilities.

Firstly, if you don't have a bolster then fold 3–4 blankets to create a bolster-like shape. Secondly make a loop in your yoga belt or a long belt or scarf about hip-distance wide.

- Start by lying flat on your back with the bolster to one side of you, close to your hips.
- Bend your knees and slide your looped belt over your legs, around mid-thigh height, so that your legs can rest into the belt. You can tighten the belt so that it supports your legs; it should feel effortless.
- Lift up your pelvis so you can slide the bolster underneath your sacrum and rest your pelvis on it. Your bolster will run horizontally across your sacrum/pelvis but not across your lower back.
- You can take your hands to the bolster and gently press the bolster away from

your head, so you feel the flesh of the back of your body lengthen away from you (see Figure 153).

• Your arms can stay down by your sides, or you can elevate them above your head to increase the opening of the front of your body and armpits.

You can also firm your belly and lengthen out one leg. If this feels okay, then explore what it feels like to lengthen both legs out. If it changes the shape of your neutral spine or you feel it in your lower back, just stretch out one leg at a time. Keep your feet flexed as if there was an imaginary wall at the end of your mat. I love this pose as it feels like it is the opposite of sitting (see Figure 154).

Variation with chair

• Place a chair at the foot end of your mat with the seat facing in.
• Place your bolster widthways across your mat.
• Sit on your bolster facing the chair.
• Place a yoga belt across your thighs and swing your legs onto the chair so that your calves rest on the chair seat.
• Lie back onto the mat, adjusting the bolster so that it is across your pelvis and not your lower back.
• Lengthen your arms away from your body. You can keep them in a T-shape or bend your elbows so that your arms are in a 'W' or 'goalpost' shape (see Figure 155).

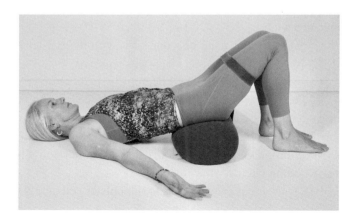

Figure 153
Supported bridge pose

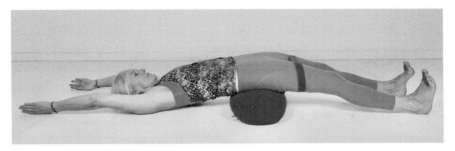

Figure 154 Releasing hip flexors

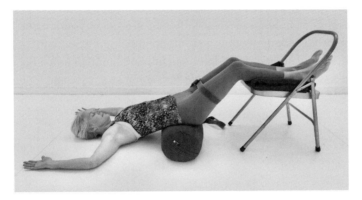

Figure 155 Legs over chair restorative option

ⓒ 5 minutes to calm and ground

Supported child's pose

This pose is good for constipation as the shape of the pose allows us to soften and release any holding in the abdomen. This forward-fold also brings our breath awareness into the back of the body. Energetically, forward-folds help to foster a sense of calm, and our awareness is drawn inwards rather than to our normal outward focus.

This pose can be done over a bolster or with a pile of folded blankets instead; be generous with the blankets as you may need them to support you in this pose. If your knees are not happy being folded like this, then you can put blankets at the backs of your legs to give yourself more space at the knees (see Figure 156).

If it is not comfortable to put pressure on your breasts or chest area, you can use blankets on top of your bolster to create space for your breasts so that there is no pain lying on the front of your body. You can be creative and use the props to mould around your body and elevate where you need a little lift. If you feel that your hips are tight, then maybe make some more space beneath your pelvis and thighs by adding a blanket here or elevate the bolster by placing something underneath it.

To keep the neutral curve of your neck, place some support underneath your forehead. If you are turning your face to one side, then turn your gaze to the other side halfway through your restorative time in order to keep balance in your neck.

Allow your shoulder blades to soften down to the floor. You should feel gravity drawing them away from each other. Relax your arms and just settle and surrender and let any clenching or holding in your belly be released as you breathe. Breathe wide into the back of your body feeling your clothing being moved with your breath and, as you exhale, you can melt down into your support and feel how you are being held. You don't need to hold onto any tension. You can just release and let go.

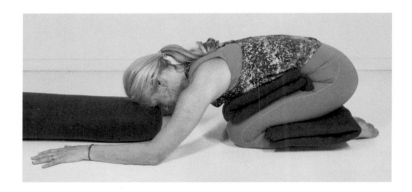

Figure 156 Supported child's pose

18

Creating a sequence

Ⓔ Ⓙ **Begin your day – awakening**

Try setting your alarm for 15 minutes before you usually get up.
- Start with a few energising breaths from Chapter 12: Breathing practices.
- Then spend 5 minutes seated, opening your feet and spine (see Chapter 15, Figures 74–91 and pages 184–185).
- Then spend 5 minutes hip opening, standing (see Chapter 16, Figures 122–126, 131–134 and 136 and page 186).
- Finally, spend 5 minutes opening your face, jaw neck and shoulders (see Chapter 15, Figures 92–107 and pages 187–188).

Opening feet and mobilising spine

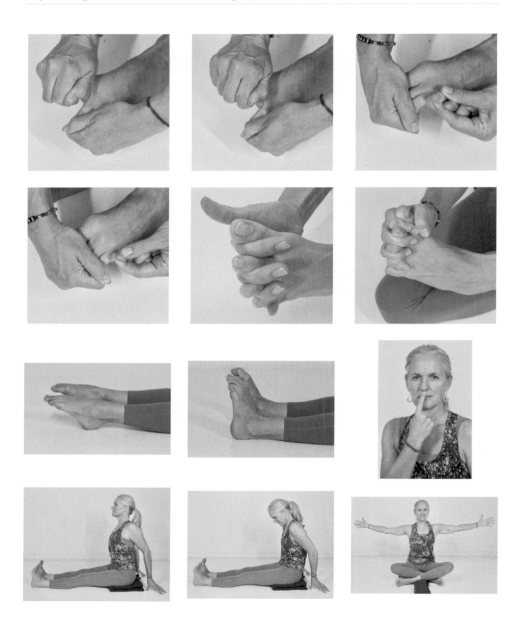

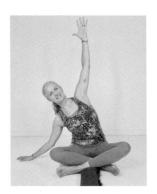
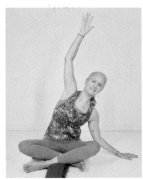
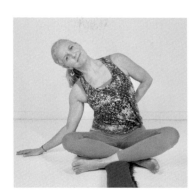

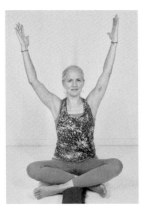
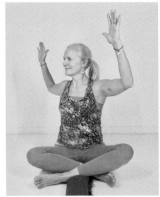
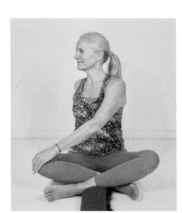

Hip opening

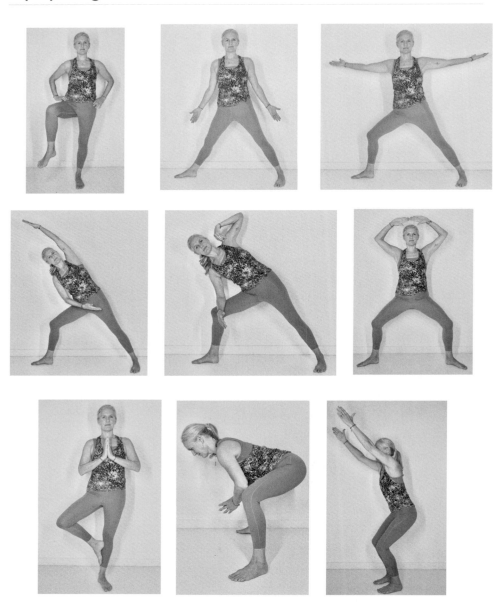

Opening face, jaw, neck and shoulders

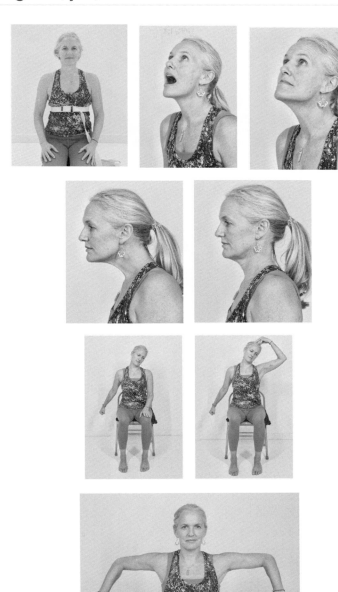

Opening face, jaw, neck and shoulders Cont'd

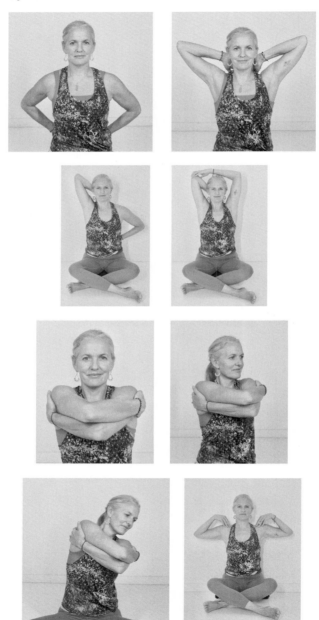

Ⓒ Ⓛ Ⓙ End your day – preparing for sleep

Start this routine by yawning to release any tension held in your mouth and jaw.

- Imagine a clock in front of you. Without moving your head, look up to 12 o'clock, then circle your eyes round to 1, 2, 3, 4, 5, and 6 o'clock, then continue circling your eyes to 7, 8, 9, 10, 11 o'clock and come back to 12. Repeat 3–4 more times.
- Practise some diaphragmatic breathing (see Chapter 5, Figure 2, page 39) or some alternate nostril breathing, breathing into the left nostril and out of the right nostril (see Figures 17 and 18, page 90 and below).
- Next, spend 5 minutes to digest (see Chapter 14, Figures 25–39 repeated on page 190).
- Next, spend 5 minutes to lubricate and flow (see Chapter 14, Figures 56–71 repeated on page 191).
- Cross your arms and place your hands into your armpits. Breathe into your hands.
- Finish with either 'legs up the wall' (see Figure 150, page 176 and repeated on page 192) or 'child's pose' (see Figure 156, page 182).
- Add in humming breath (see page 91) if you find your mind is still busy.

Alternate nostril breathing

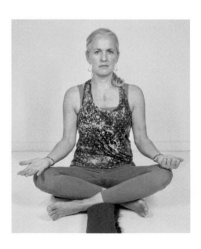 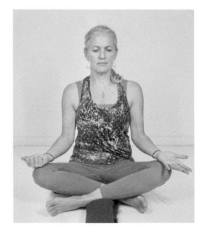

Digest

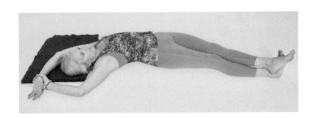
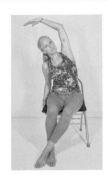
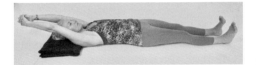
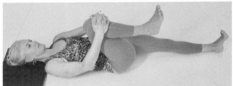
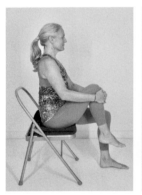
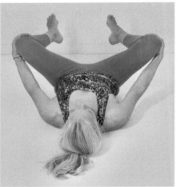
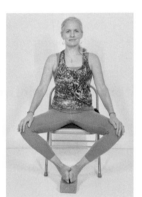
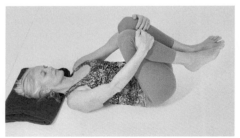

Lubricate and flow

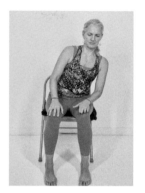

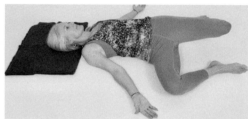

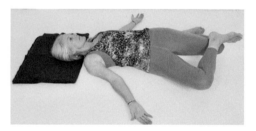

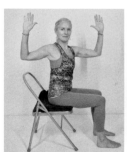 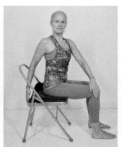 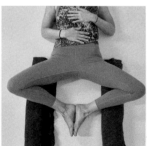 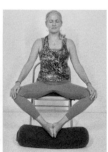

Lubricate and flow, Cont'd

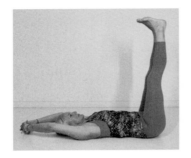 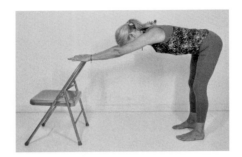

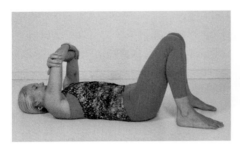 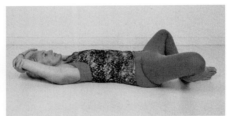

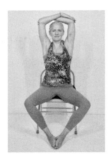 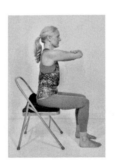

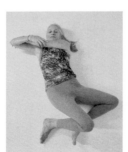 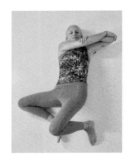

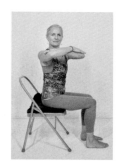

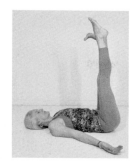

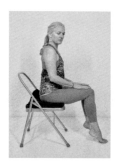

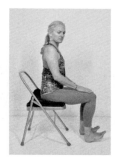

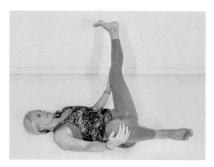

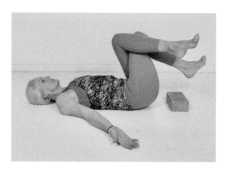

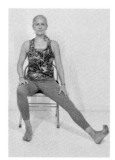

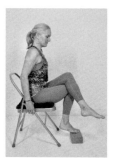

End your practice

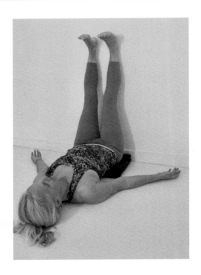

References

Chapter 1: Taking control 5 minutes at a time

1. Cramer H, Lauche R, Klose P, Lange S, Langhorst J, Dobos GJ. Yoga for improving health-related quality of life, mental health and cancer-related symptoms in women diagnosed with breast cancer. *Cochrane Database of Systematic Reviews* 2017; 1(1). Available at: https://doi-org/10.1002/14651858.CD010802.pub2
2. NYU Langone Health/NYU School of Medicine. Yoga shown to improve anxiety, study shows. *ScienceDaily* 12 August 2020. Available at: www.sciencedaily.com/releases/2020/08/200812144124.htm (Accessed: 21 October 2022).
3. Fishman LM. Yoga for osteoporosis - a pilot study. *Topics in Geriatric Rehabilitation* 2009; 25(3): 244–250. Available at: https://doi-org/10.1097/TGR.0b013e3181b02dd6
4. Wang Y, Lu S, Wang R, Jiang P, Rao F, Wang B, Zhu Y, Hu Y, Zhu J. Integrative effect of yoga practice in patients with knee arthritis: a PRISMA-compliant meta-analysis. *Medicine (Baltimore)* 2018; 97(31): e11742. Available at: https://doi-org/10.1097/MD.0000000000011742
5. Sivaramakrishnan D, Fitzsimons C, Kelly P, Ludwig K, Mutrie N, Saunders DH, Baker G The effects of yoga compared to active and inactive controls on physical function and health related quality of life in older adults- systematic review and meta-analysis of randomised controlled trials', *Int J Behav Nutr Phys Act* 2019; 16(1): 33. Available at: https://doi-org/10.1186/s12966-019-0789-2
6. Amin DJ, Goodman M. The effects of selected asanas in Iyengar yoga on flexibility: pilot study. *J Bodyw Mov Ther* 2014; 18(3): 399–404. Available at: https://doi-org/10.1016/j.jbmt.2013.11.008
7. Djalilova DM, Schulz PS, Berger AM, Case AJ, Kupzyk KA, Ross AC. Impact of yoga on inflammatory biomarkers: a systematic review. *Biological Research For Nursing* 2019; 21(2): 198–209. Available at: https://doi –org/10.1177/1099800418820162
8. Sivaramakrishnan D, Fitzsimons C, Kelly P, Ludwig K, Mutrie N, Saunders

DH, Baker G. The effects of yoga compared to active and inactive controls on physical function and health related quality of life in older adults – systematic review and meta-analysis of randomised controlled trials', *Int J Behav Nutr Phys Act* 2019; 16(1): 33. Available at: https://doi-org/10.1186/s12966-019-0789-2

9. Vardar Yağlı N, Şener G, Arıkan H, et al. Do yoga and aerobic exercise training have impact on functional capacity, fatigue, peripheral muscle strength, and quality of life in breast cancer survivors? *Integrative Cancer Therapies* 2015; 14(2):125–132. Available at: https//doi-org/10.1177/1534735414565699

10. Russell N, Daniels B, Smoot B, Allen D. Effects of yoga on quality of life and pain in women with chronic pelvic pain: systematic review and meta-analysis. *Journal of Women's Health Physical Therapy* 2019; 43(3): 144–154. Available at: https//doi-org/10.1097/JWH.0000000000000135

11. Falkenberg RI, Eising C, Peters ML. Yoga and immune system functioning: a systematic review of randomized controlled trials. *J Behav Med* 2018; 41(4): 467–482. Available at: https://doi-org/10.1007/s10865-018-9914-y

12. Institute of Science and Technology Austria. Neuroscientists discover new learning rule for pattern completion. *ScienceDaily* 13 May 2016. Available at: www.sciencedaily.com/releases/2016/05/160513111839.htm

13. van Aalst J, Ceccarini J, Demyttenaere K, Sunaert S, Van Laere K. What has neuroimaging taught us on the neurobiology of yoga? A review. *Front Integr Neurosci* 2020; 14: 34. Available at: https://doi-org/10.3389/fnint.2020.00034

14. Dispenza J. *You are the placebo*. London: Hay House UK; 2012.

15. Brown M. *The presence process: a healing journey into present moment awareness*. New York, NY: Beaufort Books; 2005.

16. Weil A. *Spontaneous healing: how to discover and enhance your body's natural ability to maintain and heal itself*. London: Sphere; 1996.

17. Servan-Shreiber D. *Anticancer: a new way of life*. London: Michael Joseph; 2011.

Chapter 2: Union – creating a sense of wholeness to allow body to repair

18. Faulds D. *Go in and in: poems from the heart of yoga*. Peaceable Kingdom Books; 2002.

19. Levine PA. *Walking the tiger: healing trauma: the innate capacity to transform overwhelming experiences*. Berkeley, CA: North Atlantic Books; 1997.

20. Adi Shankaracharya, Madhava, Alladi Mahadeva Sastri. *The Taittiriya – Upanishad*. Andesite Press; 2017. Available at: www.goodreads.com/book/show/43948726-the-taittiriya-upanishad (Accessed: 22 November 2022).

21. Pert C. *Molecules of emotion: why you feel the way you feel*. London, UK: Simon and Schuster; 1999.

22. Minford E. 'E=mc2: Everything is energy - why do we continue to ignore the energetic truth? Universal Medicine 2000.
    Available at: www.universalmedicine.co.uk/articles/emc2-everything-energy-why-do-we-continue-ignore-energetic-truth (Accessed: 21 October 2022).

23. Rodenburg P. *Presence – how to use positive energy for success in every situation*. London: Penguin; 2009.

24. Hamasaki H. Effects of diaphragmatic breathing on health: a narrative review. *Medicines (Basel)* 2020; 7(10).
    Available at: https//doi-org/10.3390/medicines7100065

25. Taylor JB. *My stroke of insight: a brain scientist's personal journey*. London: Hodder & Stoughton; 2008.

26. Hanh TN. *Understanding our mind*. Berkeley, CA: Parallax Press; 2021.
    Available at: https://plumvillage.org/articles/the-mind-as-a-gardener/ (Accessed: 22 October 2022).

27. Turner KA. *Radical remission, surviving cancer against all odds*. Boulder, CO: Bravo Books; 2015.

Chapter 3: Energetics of the body

28. Swami Muktibodhananda. *Hatha yoga pradipika*. Munger, Bihar, India: Yoga Publications Trust; 2011.

29. Rowden A. What is a normal respiratory rate based on your age? *Medical News Today* 21 December 2021. Available at:
    www.medicalnewstoday.com/articles/324409 (Accessed: 22 October 2022).

30. Swami Niranjanananda Saraswati. *Prana and pranayama*. Munger, Bihar, India: Yoga Publications Trust; 2016.

31. Sovik R. *Moving inward: the journey to meditation*. Honesdale, PA: Himalyan Institute Press; 2006.

32. Swami Satyananda Saraswati and Swami Niranjanananda. *Prana Vidya*. Munger, Bihar, India: Yoga Publications Trust; 2013.

Chapter 4: Love is everything

33. Wet Wet Wet. *Love is all around us*. London: The Precious Organisation; 1994.
34. Beatles. *All you need is love*. London: Olympic Sound and EMI; 1967.
35. Fox V. *Yoga for cancer: A–Z of C*. London: Hammersmith Press; 2022.

Chapter 5: Domes and their role in the health of our body

36. Price N. *Inspirational breathing*. Available at: www.inspirationalbreathing.com/ (Accessed: 22 October 2022).
37. Bordoni B, Zanier E. (2013) 'Anatomic connections of the diaphragm: influence of respiration on the body system. *J Multidiscip Healthc* 2013; 6: 281–291. Available at: https://doi-org/10.2147/JMDH.S45443
38. Howard L. *Pelvic liberation using: yoga, self-inquiry, and breath awareness for pelvic health*. London: Leslie Howard Yoga; 2017: p. 50.

Chapter 6: Union and the immune system

39. Quaresma JAS. Organization of the skin immune system and compartmentalized immune responses in infectious diseases. *Clin Microbiol Rev* 2019; 32(4): e00034–18. Available at: https://doi-org/10.1128/CMR.00034-18
40. Morris, N. This 'circulation boosting' home workout could improve your immune system. *Metro* 13 November 2020. Available at: https://metro.co.uk/2020/11/13/this-circulation-boosting-home-workout-could-improve-immune-system-13588998/ (Accessed: 23 October 2022).
41. Panjeta E, Panjeta M, Derviševic A, Ćorić J. Effect of yoga exercise on circulatory system. *J Yoga & Physio* 2019; 8(1): 555726. Available at: https://doi-org/10.19080/JYP.2019.08.555726
42. Woodyard C. Exploring the therapeutic effects of yoga and its ability to increase quality of life. *Int J Yoga* 2011; 4(2): 49–54. Available at: http://doi-org/10.4103/0973-6131.85485
43. Nestor J. *Breath: the new science of a lost art*. New York (NY): Riverhead Books; 2020.

44. University of California – Los Angeles. Study shows how serotonin and a popular anti-depressant affect the gut's microbiota. *ScienceDaily* 6 September 2019. Available at: www.sciencedaily.com/releases/2019/09/190906092809.htm

45. Wu H-J, Wu E. The role of gut microbiota in immune homeostasis and autoimmunity. *Gut Microbes* 2012; 3: 4–14.
Available at: https://doi.org/10.4161/gmic.19320

46. Fields H. The gut: where bacteria and immune system meet', *John Hopkins Medicine* 2015. Available at: www.hopkinsmedicine.org/research/advancements-in-research/fundamentals/in-depth/the-gut-where-bacteria-and-immune-system-meet (Accessed: 23 October 2022).

47. Cancer Research UK. *What are the benefits of exercise?* 2021. Available at: www.cancerresearchuk.org/about-cancer/causes-of-cancer/physical-activity-and-cancer/what-are-the-benefits-of-exercise (Accessed: 23 October 2022).

48. The Lymphoedema Support Network (LSN). *What is lymphoedema?* 2019. Available at: www.lymphoedema.org/information/what-is-lymphoedema/ (Accessed: 23 October 2022).

49. Suami H, Koelmeyer L, Mackie H, Boyages J. Patterns of lymphatic drainage after axillary node dissection impact arm lymphoedema severity: a review of animal and clinical imaging studies. *Surg Oncol* 2018; 27(4): 743–750. Available at: https://doi-org/10.1016/j.suronc.2018.10.006

50. Nelson TS, Nepiyushchikh Z, Hooks JST, et al. Lymphatic remodelling in response to lymphatic injury in the hind limbs of sheep', *Nat Biomed Eng* 2020; 4: 649–661. Available at: https://doi.org/10.1038/s41551-019-0493-1

51. University of Georgia (2020) Growing back the lymph system. *Newswise* 8 May 2020. Available at: www.newswise.com/articles/growing-back-the-lymph-system (Accessed: 23 October 2022).

52. Cancer Research UK. *Physical activity and cancer*. Available at: www.cancerresearchuk.org/about-cancer/causes-of-cancer/physical-activity-and-cancer/what-are-the-benefits-of-exercise (Accessed: 23 October 2022).

Chapter 7: The immune system and stress

53. Mariotti A. The effects of chronic stress on health: new insights into the molecular mechanisms of brain-body communication. *Future Sci OA* 2015; 1(3): FSO23. Available at: https://doi-org/10.4155/fso.15.21

54. Patel JD. What is scanxiety? how people with cancer and survivors can cope', *Cancer.net* 28 October 2021. Available at: www.cancer.net/blog/2021-10/what-scanxiety-how-people-with-cancer-and-survivors-can-cope (Accessed: 23 October 2022).

55. Porges SW. *Polyvagal theory*. 2022. Available at: www.stephenporges.com/ (Accessed: 23 October 2022).

56. van der Kolk, B. *The body keeps the score: mind, brain and body in the transformation of trauma*. London: Allen Lane; 2014.

57. Mind *Information and support* 2022. Available at: www.mind.org.uk/information-support/ (Accessed: 23 October 2022).

58. West, S.G. (2003) *Growing an inch*. Carver, MN: Lexington Marshall Publishing.

59. Sarkar DK, Murugan S, Zhang C, Boyadjieva N. Regulation of cancer progression by β-endorphin neuron. *Cancer Res* 2012; 72(4): 836–840. Available at: https://doi-org/10.1158/0008-5472.CAN-11-3292

Chapter 8: Building strength, bones and muscles

60. Lu YH, Rosner B, Chang G, Fishman LM. Twelve-minute daily yoga regimen reverses osteoporotic bone loss', *Top Geriatr Rehabil* 2016; 32(2): 81–87. Available at: https://doi-org/10.1097/TGR.0000000000000085

61. NHS *Osteoporosis* 2022. Available at: www.nhs.uk/conditions/osteoporosis/causes/ (Accessed: 25 March 2022).

62. Ji MX, Yu Q. (2015) Primary osteoporosis in postmenopausal women. *Chronic Dis Transl Med* 2015; 1(1): 9–13. Available at: http://doi-org/10.1016/j.cdtm.2015.02.006

63. International Osteoporosis Foundation (IOF) *Exercise for individuals with osteoporosis* 2022. Available at: www.osteoporosis.foundation/health-professionals/prevention/exercise/exercise-individuals-with-osteoporosis (Accessed: 26 March 2022).

64. McGonigle A. *Supporting yoga students with common injuries and conditions: a handbook for teachers and trainees*. London: Singing Dragon; 2021.

65. Schnell S, Friedman SM, Mendelson DA, Bingham KW, Kates SL. The 1-year mortality of patients treated in a hip fracture program for elders. *Geriatr Orthop Surg Rehabil* 2010; 1(1): 6–14.

Available at: https://doi-org/10.1177/2151458510378105

66. Lisk R, Yeong K.(2014) 'Reducing mortality from hip fractures: a systematic quality improvement programme. *BMJ Qual Improv Rep* 2014; 3(1). Available at: https://doi-org/10.1136/bmjquality.u205006.w2103

67. Mathis SL, Farley RS, Fuller DK, Jetton AE, Caputo JL. (2013) The relationship between cortisol and bone mineral density in competitive male cyclists', *J Sports Med (Hindawi Publ Corp)* 2013; 2013: Article: 896821. Available at: https://doi-org/10.1155/2013/896821

68. Katuri KK, Dasari AB, Kurapati S, Vinnakota NR, Bollepalli AC, Dhulipalla R. Association of yoga practice and serum cortisol levels in chronic periodontitis patients with stress-related anxiety and depression. *J Int Soc Prev Community Dent* 2016; 6(1): 7–14. Available at: https://doi/10.4103/2231-0762.175404

69. Hamilton D. *Can kindness boost the immune system?* 24 July 2018. Available at: https://drdavidhamilton.com/can-kindness-boost-the-immune-system/ (Accessed: 24 October 2022).

70. Ornish D. *Ornish lifestyle medicine* 2022. Available at: www.ornish.com/ (Accessed: 24 October 2022).

71. Clark BC, Mahato NK, Nakazawa M, Law TD, Thomas JS. The power of the mind: the cortex as a critical determinant of muscle strength/weakness. *J Neurophysiol* 2014; 112(12): 3219–3226. Available at: https://doi-org/10.1152/jn.00386.2014

72. Yao WX, Ranganathan VK, Allexandre D, Siemionow V, Yue GH. Kinesthetic imagery training of forceful muscle contractions increases brain signal and muscle strength. *Front Hum Neurosci* 2013; 7: 561. Available at: https://doi-org/10.3389/fnhum.2013.00561

73. Reiser M, Büsch D, Munzert J. Strength gains by motor imagery with different ratios of physical to mental practice. *Frontiers in Psychology* 2011; 2(194). Available at: https://doi-org/10.3389/fpsyg.2011.00194

74. Helm F, Marinovic W, Krüger B, Munzert J, Riek S. Corticospinal excitability during imagined and observed dynamic force production tasks: effortfulness matters. *Neuroscience* 2015; 290: 398–405. Available at: https://doi-org/10.1016/j.neuroscience.2015.01.050

Chapter 9: Starting to practise

75. Swami Satchidananda Saraswati. *Yoga sutras of Patanjali*. Buckingham, VA: Integral Yoga Publications; 2012.
76. Farhi D. *Bringing yoga to life: the everyday practice of enlightened living*. London: HarperCollins; 2008.

Chapter 10: Mudras – hand gestures

77. Hirschi G. *Mudras: yoga in your hands*. London: Coronet; 2016: p. 90.
78. Hirschi G. *Mudras: yoga in your hands*. London: Coronet; 2016: p. 102.

Chapter 11: Mantras to anchor

79. Nepo M. *Coming up for air* 2020. Available at: https://community.thriveglobal.com/growing-in-place-with-mark-nepo-6/ (Accessed: 22 November 2022).
80. Swami Satyananda Saraswati and Swami Niranjanananda. *Prana Vidya*. Munger, Bihar, India: Yoga Publications Trust; 2013.
81. Goldsby, T.L., Goldsby, M.E., McWalters, M. and Mills, P.J. Effects of singing bowl sound meditation on mood, tension, and well-being: an observational study. *J Evid Based Complementary Altern Med* 2017; 22(3): 401–406. Available at: https://doi-org/10.1177/2156587216668109
82. Porges S. *The polyvagal theory: neurophysiological foundations of emotions, attachment, communication and self-regulation*. New York (NY): WW Norton & Co; 2011.
83. Sovik R. *Moving inward: the journey to meditation*. Honesdale, PA: Himalyan Institute Press; 2006.
84. Ashley-Farrand T. *Healing mantras: using sound affirmations for personal power, creativity, and healing*. New York (NY): Ballantine Books Inc; 1999.

Chapter 12: Breathing practices

85. Swami Mukundananda (2014) *The Bhagavad Gita* 2014. Chapter 5, Verse 27–

28. Available at: www.holy-bhagavad-gita.org/chapter/5/verse/27-28 (Accessed: 24 October 2022).

86. Swami Satchidananda Saraswati. *Yoga sutras of Patanjali.* Buckingham, VA: Integral Yoga Publications; 2012.

87. Easwaran E. (trans.) *The Bhagavad Gita.* Tomales, CA: Blue Mountain Center of Meditation; Nilgiri Press; 2007: Chapter 6, verses 19–20, p. 142.

88. Gach MR, Henning BA. *Acupressure for emotional healing: a self-care guide for trauma, stress, and common emotional imbalances: a self-care guide for trauma, stress, & common emotional imbalances.* New York (NY): Broadway Books; 2004: p. 231.

89. McKay L. *Field yoga* 2022. Available at: https://fieldyoga.com/about-field-yoga/ (Accessed: 22 November 2022).

90. Iyengar BKS. *Light on yoga: the bible of modern yoga.* New York (NY): Schocken Books; 1996: p. 139.

91. Memorial Sloan Kettering Cancer Center. *A field in motion: fighting cancer with exercise* [video] 2016. Available at: www.mskcc.org/msk-community/programs-services/cancersmart/cancersmart-live-webcast-exercise (Accessed: 24 October 2022).

92. Harvard Health Publishing. *Cancer treatments may harm the heart*, 1 August 2012. Available at: www.health.harvard.edu/heart-health/cancer-treatments-may-harm-the-heart (Accessed: 24 October 2022).

93. Bradshaw PT, Stevens J, Khankari N, Teitelbaum SL, Neugut AI, Gammon MD. Cardiovascular disease mortality among breast cancer survivors. *Epidemiology* 2016; 27(1): 6–13. Available at: https://doi-org/10.1097/EDE.0000000000000394

Chapter 15: Asana practice – seated

94. Carpenter A. *Smart flow yoga* 2020. Available at: www.smartflowyoga.com/ (Accessed: 24 October 2022).

95. Gach MR, Henning BA. *Acupressure for emotional healing: a self-care guide for trauma, stress, and common emotional imbalances: a self-care guide for trauma, stress, and common emotional imbalances.* New York (NY): Broadway Books; 2004: p. 274.

Glossary of yoga terms

Ahimsa: Ahimsa is the first of the 'eight limbs' of yoga and means 'non-harming' or 'non-violence'. Non-harming in the way we treat others and ourselves. Ahimsa is not just the absence of violence, but the presence of love.

Ajna chakra: The energetic centre associated with clarity, intuition and the power of our mind. Often called the 'third eye'.

Anahata chakra: Also known as the heart centre, this wheel of energy can be stimulated when we practise poses that open up the heart or we practise loving kindness meditations or any compassion-based kindness or heart-felt prayers that nourish our hearts.

Anandamaya kosha: Fifth layer or sheath of the koshas, the bliss body.

Annamaya kosha: First layer or sheath of the koshas, the physical or gross body.

Apana vayu: Apana is one of the energy vayus that focuses on physical downward elimination movements like defaecation, urination and menstruation to remove unwanted substances from the body.

Apana vayu mudra: A mudra focusing on downward-moving energy formed by bringing your index fingers to the base of your thumb and then bringing your ring and middle finger to the tip of the thumb.

Apanasana: Wind-relieving pose.

Asana: Posture or seat. According to Patanjali, asana is a steady and comfortable meditative pose or seat.

Aum: Said to be the primordial sound born with the universe, aum is a mantra chanted to connect to the universe and tune into our higher sense of self.

Bija: One-syllable mantras that have a particular vibration.

Brahmari breathing: Humming (buzzing bee) breathing using different sounds as you exhale to stimulate udana vayu, calm the nervous system and draw awareness inwards.

Brahmari mudra: The bee mudra is created by bringing the index finger to the base of the thumb and the tip of your thumb to the inside of your middle finger close to the fingernail. This mudra is said to help strengthen the immune system.

Chakra: A wheel or energy centre that the subtle energy of the body moves through. Each of the seven chakras is reliant on the energetic flow of the others for energy to flow freely through the body.

Garuda mudra: Supports vyana and 'activates blood flow and circulation',[78] invigorates the organs and balances energy on both sides. Hook your thumbs and place your hands onto your belly with your right hand on top of your left.

Gayatri mantra: A mantra for gratitude which gives thanks to the sun that is forever giving and never receiving, with the wish that the sun might shine through and inspire all of us.

Gomukasana: Cow-face pose: 'go' means cow, 'mukha' means face and 'asana' means seat. The arms in this position look like cow's ears.

Hakini mudra: Bringing the fingertips of each hand together like a tee pee or tent; said to be a mudra for the mind.

Ham: A one-syllable mantra relating to help cleanse or balance energy at the throat.

Ida nadi: Major energy channel that runs along the spine to the end of the left nostril and is said to be cooling and calming.

Japa: The process of repeating a mantra.

Jatharagni: Jatharagni is the digestive fire within all of us. The gut strength that helps us to digest life experiences as well as our food.

Koshas: The yoga tradition of viewing the body as multi-layered sheaths or bodies that are all linked.

Lam: A one-syllable mantra relating to the base of the spine helping to clear stuck energy in this area and to give a sense of grounding or being more connected to the earth.

Manipura chakra: This chakra relates to the area between the navel and the rib cage. Also referred to as the solar plexus chakra.

Manomaya kosha: Our mental sheath or body where we process our experiences.

Mantras: Sacred sounds that can be used as tools for meditation. 'Man' means 'mind' and 'tra' means 'to protect from', so these mantras help protect our mind. 'Tra' can also be translated as 'tool' so 'mantra' can also mean a tool for the mind.

Matangi mudra: Supports samana vayu; interlace all of the fingers except the middle fingers. Extend the middle fingers and place against each other. Then lower your hands to rest at your belly with your fingers pointing out away from the navel.

Mudras: Literally meaning 'gesture', this term can refer to a hand position, eye position or even asanas or breathing techniques.

Muladhara chakra: The root or muladhara chakra is located at the base of your spine and linked to you feeling rooted or grounded in life.

Nadis: A complex, subtle system of energy channels which flow through the body nourishing our muscles, organs and cells.

Nadi shodana: Alternate nostril breathing. 'Nadi' means channel and 'shodhana' means purification so the breathing helps to clear the channels of the subtle body. The breath can calm the mind and, depending on which nostril you are breathing into, you can also make the breathing focus more on energising.

Pingala nadi: An energy channel that runs along the spine to the end of the right nostril and is said to be warming or energising.

Prana: The vital energy or life force that flows forwards and upwards through the body, sustaining life and creation. We can influence the flow of prana through breathing techniques.

Prana mudra: A mudra to help encourage the prana or energy into the body. Bring the thumb, little and ring finger to touch on both hands.

Pranamaya kosha: Subtle layer of the body of breath or energy.

Pranayama: 'Ayama' means to stretch or extend, and 'prana' is the energy that keeps us alive. Simon Low also taught me that 'pra' means consistent, 'prana' means life force and 'ayama' means to stretch, so that pranayama is a consistent practice of breathing techniques that help the flow of prana.

Pratyahara: The fifth of the eight limbs of yoga and is often translated as withdrawal from the senses or drawing the awareness inwards as we do with pranayama. Pratyahara helps prepare us for meditation.

Sahasrara chakra: The sahasrara chakra is located at the top of the head and is also known as the crown chakra.

Samana vayu: 'Saman' means 'balanced', 'vayu' means wind and this movement of energy is active at the navel centre (manipura chakra) and supports healthy digestion of food but also experiences and memories. It works in conjunction with our digestive fire known as jatharagni.

Savasana: Final resting pose where you are relaxed but conscious. All the doing is done, and you can be a human being.

Shankh mudra: Supports udana vayu. Close your left thumb into the fingers of your right hand and then bring your right thumb to the extended fingers of your left hand. Create sounds and vibrations as you hold the hand against your sternum.

Sitali: Cooling breathing techniques using an extended curled tongue in a straw shape or the mouth in a circle shape or by sucking air through the sides of your teeth.

So ham: Mantra meaning 'I am that', 'I am connected to everyone and everything'. Reminds us of our interconnectedness.

Sukhasana: 'Sukha' means comfort, 'asana' means seat, so this cross-legged seated position is said to be an 'easy seat'.

Supta baddha konasana: A restorative pose to open up the belly and groin area. 'Supta' means 'lying supine', 'baddha' means 'bound' and 'kona' means 'angle'.

Sushumna nadi: The main energy channel running along the spinal column from the base of the spine to the top of the nostrils.

Sutras: 'Sutras' means 'threads', or short pieces of text threaded together.

Svadisthana chakra: This second chakra, also known as the sacral chakra, is located at the lower belly and pelvis.

Tadasana: The mountain pose, a grounded standing posture that helps to create a healthy alignment that you can keep throughout all the other poses or asanas.

Trikonasana: The triangle pose, an energising pose that stretches upper and lower body and strengthens core muscles.

Udana vayu: Udana vayu is one of the five winds of life force or energy known as prana. It is an ascending force that rules the throat centre and our ability to be articulate and express ourselves.

Vajra mudra: Said to stimulate circulation. Press your thumb to the side of the middle finger by the nail. Press the ring finger to the other side of the middle finger and the little finger at the side of your ring fingernail. Do this with both hands with the index fingers extended out.

Vayu: Subtle movement of energy that can be divided into five sub-energies known as vayus, which is often translated as 'winds'. Vayu comes from the root 'va' meaning 'motion' or 'flow'. The five vayus that move in different directions are prana, apana, samana, vyana and udana and, when balanced, they allow energy to move throughout the whole body.

Vijnyanamaya kosha: Our intuitive or wisdom sheath or layer of the body.

Viloma: 'Vi' means 'against' and 'loma' means 'hair', so 'viloma' means 'against the natural flow' and is a breathing technique for controlling the breath. Viloma 1 can be used to energise the body if it focuses on inhale. Viloma 2 focuses on exhale.

Viparita karani: 'Legs up the wall', a pose which is calming for the nervous system. 'Viparita' means 'inverted' and 'karani' means 'in action'. The pose helps by turning the body upside down to give it a break from its normal functioning of having to pump blood back towards the heart.

Vishuddha chakra: Also known as the throat chakra, stimulating this wheel of energy helps us to find our voice and be authentic in how we speak.

Vyana vayu: Vyana is an expansive energy that distributes energy out to the periphery of the body, the arms, legs, fingers and toes. Expanding out from the heart this all-pervading vital energy of the heart and lungs governs circulation.

Yoga: A state of union between body and mind, individual and universal awareness.

Index

abdominal (diaphragmatic) breathing, 39, 183

abdominal muscles, 105

    transverse, 38

adrenaline, 49, 50, 53

agonist–antagonist muscle pairs and static postures, 59

ahimsa, 67, **203**

ajna chakra, 27–28, **203**

alternate nostril breathing (nadi shodana), 28, 89–90, 189, **205-206**

anahata (heart centre chakra), 25–26, 29, 30, 31, **203**

anandamaya kosha, 17, **203**

anchoring (into present moment), 14, 67, 81

    mantras, 79–81

ankles, circling, 127, 132

annamaya kosha (phyical layer), 11, 13, **203**

apana vayu, 19, 21, **203**, 200

    mudras supporting, 76, 103, **203**

apanasana (wind-relieving pose), **203**

    supine downward dog, 120–121

apanasana flow, 103–106

arms

    in bear-hug rib opener, 146–147

    scarecrow, 144

asanas (postures/poses), 15, **203**

    joint-challenging, 59

    seated (floor), 131–148

    standing, 149–174

    static, 58–59, 60

    supine, 101–130

Ashley-Farrand, Thomas, 81

attention, 4, 12–13, 15

    body scan, 87

    in meditation, 97

aum, 79, 80–81, 80–81, **203**

autonomic nervous system, 39, 50–52

    see also parasympathetic nervous system; sympathetic nervous system

awakening, 183

axillary node dissection, 46

ayurveda yoga, 74

back (lower), tapping, 144

baddha konasana

    seated, 108

    supta *see* supta baddha konasana

baddha konasana flow, framed, 121–122

balance, 57–58, 166–174

    bringing energetic centres into, 28

    chair helping with, 71

    improving, 57–58

bear-hug rib opener, 146–147

bedtime practices, 183–184

bee

    the bee (brahmari mudra), 177, **204**

    buzzing bee (brahmari breathing), 91, **204**

belly (diaphragmatic) breathing, 39, 183

belts *see* straps and belts

bending, safe practice, 56–57

    see also forward-fold/bends

Bhagavad Gita, 84, 85

bicycle legs, 110–111

bija, 24, 80, **204**

blankets

    in calf release, 151

    child's pose, 181

    in legs over chair, 176

Note: Bold indicates glossary definitions. Illustrations (figures and tables) are comprehensively referred to from the text. Therefore, significant items in illustrations have only been given a page reference in the absence of their concomitant mention in the text referring to that illustration.

viparita karani with, 175–176
bliss layer (anandamaya kosha), 17, **203**
blocks/bricks, 69–70
  asymmetrical glute lifts, 114
  forward-fold, 165
  half-wide V, 126, 128
  hip opening, 149, 186
  hugging between shins, 149
  strengthening
    respiratory diaphragm, 38
    standing, 149
blood, circulation, 20, 22, 43, 77
blood cells
  red, 41, 42
  white, 42, 45–46, 49, 177
body
  layers/sheaths *see* koshas
  union between mind and, 200
body scan, 87–89
bolsters, 70
  bridge, 179–180
  supta baddha konasana, 178
bone, 55–64
  fractures *see* fractures
  strengthening, 42, 55–64
bone marrow, 42
brahmari breathing, 91, **204**
brahmari mudra, 177, **204**
brain, 5, 12, 43
  fluid surrounding, 36, 42
  gut and, 44
  stroke, 15–16, 64
brainstem and vagus, 40
breath, layer of (pranamaya kosha), 11–13, **206**
breathing (practices), 46, 83–95
  connections and, 13–14
  diaphragmatic, 39, 183
  lymphatic system and, 46
  nose *see* nose breathing
  via nose *see* nose
  reverse, 38, 39
  strap, 140
  see also exhalation; inhalation
breathing muscles
  primary, 13, 42

secondary/auxiliary, 42, 83
bricks *see* blocks
bridge/glute lifts, 112–113
  asymmetrical, 114–115
  supported, 179–180
Brown, Michael, 5
Buddhism, 16

calf
  dynamic strengthening, 152
  muscle pump, 46–47
  release, 151–152
calmness and calming, 69, 74, 90, 91, 175, 181–182
cancer
  chemotherapy, 20, 93
  fighting talk, 31–32
  lymph node removal, 46
cardiovascular system, 41–42
  see also heart
Carpenter, Annie, 131
cat-cow, 134
central nervous system, 19, 50
cerebrospinal fluid, 36, 42
cervical diaphragms, 36–37
cervical spine (neck), 36, 61
chair (incl. alternative/optional supports for poses),
  70–71
  standing poses
    dynamic calf strengthening, 152
    dynamic chair, 154
    dynamic lunge, 156
    half-moon pose, 172
    marching, 168
    trikonasana, 172
    Warrior II and side-angle pose, 160
  supine poses
    apanasana, 106
    bicycle legs, 111
    clams, 116
    crescent moon, 101–103
    downward dog, 121
    figure-of-four stretch, 117–118
    framed baddha konasana flow, 122
    framed supine twist, 124
    glute lifts (asymmetrical), 115

glute lifts (standard), 112–113
half-wide V, 127–128
legs extended to ceiling, 125
legs over chair, 128, 176–177, 180
twists to stimulate samana vayu, 108
see also sitting
chair pose, imaginary, 165
chakras, 12, 24–28, **204**
1st (muladhara chakra), 24, **205**
2nd (svadisthana chakra), 25, **207**
3rd (manipura chakra), 25, **205**
4th (anahata chakra; heart centre), 25–26, 30, 31, **203**
5th (vishuddha chakra), 26–27, **208**
6th (ajna chakra), 27–28, **203**
7th (sahasrara chakra), 28, **206**
chanting, 80
see also mantras
chemotherapy, 20, 93
chest opening/release, 166
with strap, 154
see also front body
child pose, supported, 181–182
children, finding time away from, 68, 69
circling
ankles, 127, 132
body (while seated), 105
knees, 105, 158
shoulder/elbows, 148
toes, 132
tongue, 94–95
circulation of blood, 20, 22, 43, 77
clams, 115–116
coccyx, 61, 62
awareness, 62
collarbones, tapping, 74
compassion, 25, 32, 64, 67, 100
connection(s), 32–33
between body layers, 17
breath aiding, 13–14
loss, 11

domes, 37
to foundations (grounding), 75, 149
see also grounding; union
connective tissue, 12
domes and, 37, 38
see also fascia
control, loss of and taking, 1–8
cooling breathing (sitali), 94–95, **207**
cortisol, 49, 50, 53, 61
cow-face pose (gomukasana), 145, **204**
cow pose (seated), 134
cramping, 134
cranial diaphragm, 36
crescent moon *see* half-moon
crown (sahasrara) chakra, 28, **206**

daily practice
creating a safe space to, 68–69
making time for, 3–4, 7–8, 65
sequences, 183–184
diaphragm(s), domes and, 35–40
cervical, 36–37
cranial, 36
pelvic, 37, 83
respiratory *see* respiratory diaphragm
diaphragmatic breathing, 39, 183
digestion, 5-minute, 101–102, 190
digestive system, 44–45, 50
disconnection in trauma, 11, 51
domes *see* diaphragms and domes
downward dog/apanasana, supine, 120–121
dynamic movements
calf strengthening, 152
chair, 153–154
Warrior I, 155-157
Warrior II, 159–162

elbows, circling, 148
energy, 19–28
centres of *see* chakras
channels *see* nadis

Note: Bold indicates glossary definitions. Illustrations (figures and tables) are comprehensively referred to from the text. Therefore, significant items in illustrations have only been given a page reference in the absence of their concomitant mention in the text referring to that illustration.

layer of (pranamaya kosha), 11–13, **203**

practices giving feelings of, 90, 92–94, 175–177

vital *see* prana

enteric nervous system, 44, 50

exhalation (breathing out), 83–84

apana vayu and, 21

in diaphragm strengthening, 38

extension (pointing)

feet, 133

spine, 62, 63

face

forward and back movements, 141–143

mirroring others' facial expressions, 53–54

opening, 187

face down lying breathing practice, 38–39

Farhi, Donna, 69

fascia, 12, 47

Faulds, Danna (poet), 9

feet

connecting to foundations, 149

cramping, 134

extending, 125

flexing, 125, 180

lubricating, 131–139

opening up, 131–133, 184

see also ankle; heels; sole; toes

fight or flight/flee response, 25, 32, 39, 40, 44, 49, 50, 51

fighting talk, 31–32

figure-of-four stretch, 117–119

flexion

foot, 125, 180

hip, 56

spine, 62, 63

toes, 133

flexors, hip, release, 179, 181

foot *see* feet

forward-fold/bends, 56, 91

horse stance to, 165

in supported child's pose, 181

foundations, connecting to (grounding) grounding, 74, 75, 149

fractures

hip, 58

spinal, 56

framed baddha konasana flow, 121–122

framed supine twist, 123–124

freeze response, 49, 51

front body, releasing tension, 179–180

see also chest

garuda mudra, 77, **204**

gastrointestinal (digestive) system, 44–45, 50

gate opening, 158

gayatri mantra, 79, 81, **204**

gestures *see* mudras

glute lifts see bridge/glute lifts

goalpost twists, 138

gomukasana, 145, **204**

gongs, 80

gratitude, 32

mantra, 81, 196

gravity and lymphatic system, 47

grounding (connecting to foundations), 74, 75, 149

gut (digestive system), 44–45, 50

hakini mudra, 73, **204**

half-moon (crescent moon) pose, 172–174

with chair support, 172–174

supine, 101–103

half-wide V, 126–128

ham, 27, 79, **204**

so ham, 79, 81, **204**

Hamilton, David, 64

hamstring release, 59, 129

hand gestures *see* mudras

hanging out in the joints, 60

Hatha Yoga Pradipika, 19

healing, meaning, 6

heart, 41

fibrous sac (pericardium), 38

focus on, 99–100

meditation focusing on, 99–100

heart centre (anahata chakra), 25–26, 29, 30, 31, **203**

Hebb's law, 5

heels

bridge/glute lifts on, 112, 114

drags (seated), 115

raises

seated, 125
standing, 152
hip, 158–165
flexion, 56
flexor release, 179, 181
fractures, 58
opening, 158–165, 186
horse stance
to forward-fold, 134
to tree, 163–164
Howard, Leslie, 37
hugging *see* bear-hug rib opener; knees; legs
humming, 23, 79, 80, 91, 154, 159, 177, 184

I *see* self and I
ida nadi, 12, 19, 27, **204**
imagery, kinaesthetic, 64
immune system, 41–54
anana vayu and, 21
gut, 44
musculoskeletal system and, 42
nervous system and, 43, 49–52
stress and, 49–54
union and, 41–47
yoga and, 47
inactivity, periods of, 55
inguinal node clearance, 46
inhalation (breathing in), 83–84
apana vayu and, 21
in diaphragm strengthening, 38
intention (for practice), creating, 67–68
intuitive layer of body (vijnyanamaya kosha), 16–17,
208
Iyengar, BKS, 91

japa, 79, **205**
Jatharagni, 22, 140, **205**, 206
jaw, 88, 99
opening, 187
release under, 141
jiva, 25
joint(s), 59

challenging poses, 59
5-minute joint space, 98–99
hanging out in, 60
lubrication *see* lubrication
sounds from, 58

kinaesthetic imagery, 64
kindness (being kind), 26, 31, 64, 67
knees
bent
in apanasana, 105
in bicycle legs, 110
in savasana, 86, 87, **206**
circling, 105, 158
hugging
in apanasana, 103, 120
in marching, 170
koshas (five layers/sheaths), 6, **205**
anandamaya kosha, 17, **203**
annamaya kosha, 11, **203**
interconnectiveness, 17
manomaya kosha, 14–16, **205**
pranamaya kosha, 11–14, **206**
vijnyanamaya kosha, 16, **208**
kundalini yoga, 24

lam, 24, **205**
layers (the five) *see* koshas
legs
bicycle, 110–111
extended to ceiling, 125
hugging bricks between shins, 149
over chair, 128, 176–177, 180
side lying legs 90 degrees, 115
up wall *see* viparita karani; wall support
see also ankle; calf; feet; standing; thigh; toes
Levine, Peter, 10, 52
life, pulse of, 19, 32, 100
life force *see* prana
light, repairing, 97–98
love, 31
lubrication (and flow), 59, 120–121, 191

Note: Bold indicates glossary definitions. Illustrations (figures and tables) are comprehensively referred to from the text. Therefore, significant items in illustrations have only been given a page reference in the absence of their concomitant mention in the text referring to that illustration.

feet and spine, 131–139, 184
    lymph node removal and, 47
lumbar spine, 61, 62
    awareness, 62
lunge, dynamic, 155–156
lying down *see* face down lying breathing practice;
        side lying leg 90 degrees; supine practices
lymph (fluid), 23, 45, 47, 177
lymph nodes (lymph glands), 45
    removal, 46, 47
lymph vessels, 45, 46, 47
lymphatic system, 45–47, 66, 125, 178
lymphocytes (white blood cells), 42, 45–46, 49, 177
lymphoedema, 46, 47, 69

McGonigle, Andrew, 57
McKay, Louisa, 89
manipura chakra, 25, **205**, 198
manomaya kosha, 14–16, **205**
mantras, 13, 79–81, **205**
    anchoring, 79–81
    gayatri mantra, 79, 81, **204**
    sounds in, 23, 79–81
    universal, 80–81
marching, 167–171
mat(s), 68, 69
matangi mudra, 76, **205**
meditation, 97–100
microbiome (gut), 44
mind
    as layer of body (manomaya kosha), 14–16, **205**
    quietening, 14, 15, 16, 28, 30, 57
    union between body and, 200
mindful practice, 17, 57–58
mirror neurons, 53
motion *see* movement
mountain pose *see* tadasana
mouth, tongue circling, 94–95
movement (motion), 58–59
    dynamic *see* dynamic movements
    lymphatic system and, 46
mudras (hand gestures), 13, 73–78
    apana vayu mudra, 76, 103, **203**
    brahmari mudra, 177, **204**
    energy-supporting (prana mudra), 75, 92, **206**

garuda mudra, 77, **204**
hakini mudra, 73, **204**
matangi mudra, 76, **205**
shankh mudra, 78, **206**
vajra mudra, 77, **208**
muladhara chakra, 24, **205**
muscles
    abdominal *see* abdominal muscles
    opposing, static postures and, 59
    pumps, lymphatic system and, 46–47
    respiratory *see* breathing muscles
    strengthening, 42, 55–64
        respiratory diaphragm, 38–39
        visualising, 64
    stretching *see* stretching
musculoskeletal system and immunity, 42

nadi(s) (energy channels), 12, **205**
    ida nadi, 12, 19, 27, **204**
    pingala nadi, 12, 19, 27, **206**
    sushumna nadi, 12, 19, **207**
nadi shodana, 28, 89–90, **205-206**
natural killer cells, 45, 49
neck
    opening/release, 136, 140, 142, 143, 166, 187-188
    spine in (cervical spine), 36, 61
    strengthening, 110
    tapping, 144, 145
Nepo, Mark, 79
nerve, pulses/impulses, 12, 22, 23, 126
nerve cells (neurons)
    firing and wiring together, 5
    gut, 44
    mirror neurons, 53
nervous system
    autonomic *see* autonomic nervous system
    central, 19, 50
    enteric, 44, 50
    immune system and, 43, 49–52
    peripheral, 43, 50
neurons *see* nerve cells
neuropathy, peripheral, 43
nitric oxide, 53
nose (nostril) breathing, 42–43, 84–85
    alternate (nadi shodana), 28, 89–90, 189 **205-206**

now *see* present moment

om, 28
opening feet, 184
Ornish, Dean, 64
osteoporosis., 55, 56, 58

parasympathetic nervous system, 21, 39, 44–45, 50,
    51–52, 91
    digestion and, 44–45
    mantras and, 80, 81
Patanjali's Yoga Sutras, 85
pelvic diaphragm, 37, 83
pelvic tilt, 63
pericardium, 38
peripheral nervous system, 43, 50
peripheral neuropathy, 43
Pert, Candace, 11
physical layer (annamaya kosha), 11, 13, **203**
pingala nadi, 12, 19, 27, **206**
Porges, Stephen, 51
prana (life force/vital energy), 12, 13, 19, 20–21, 22,
    79, **206**
    mudras supporting, 75, 92, **206**
prana vayu, 19–21, **208**
pranamaya kosha, 11–14, **206**
pranayama, 22, **206**
pratyahara, 30, **206**
present moment (right now), 10, 13, 15, 21, 30, 33, 57,
    81, 85, 87, 91, 100
    anchoring into *see* anchoring
Price, Nicola, 36
prone breathing practice, 38–39
props, 69–71
pubic bone, 62, 159, 161
pulse of life, 19, 32, 100

ram, 25
red blood cells, 41, 42
repetitions, 5
respiratory diaphragm, 13, 35–36

breathing practices and, 38, 83, 85, 183
restorative practices and, 178
strengthening, 38–39
vagus and, 40
respiratory system, 42–43
rest, 61
    and digest, 21, 39, 40, 51, 61, 91, 175, 190
restorative practices, 175–184
    following supine poses, 128
    power, 2, 61
reverse breathing, 38, 39
rib opener, 146–147
root (muladhara), 24, **205**
rotations, 56
    in scarecrow arms, 144, 145
Rumi (poet), 16

sacral chakra (svadisthana), 25, **207**
sacral plexus (manipura) chakra, 25, **205, 206**
sacrum, 25, 61, 62, 179
    awareness, 62
safety
    bending and twisting, 56–57
    creating a safe space to repair, 68–69
sahasrara chakra, 28, **206**
samana vayu, 19, 22, 103, **206**, 200
    mudras supporting, 76
    twists to stimulate, 106–107
savasana, 86, 87, **206**
scar tissue release, 12, 23, 47
scarecrow arms, 144
seated *see* chair; sitting
seaweed feet, 133
self and I, 10
    awareness of, 10
Servan-Shreiber, D., 7
shankh mudra, 78, **206**
sheaths (the five) *see* koshas
shoulders, 142, 144, 145, 146, 178
    circles, 148
    opening, 187-188

Note: Bold indicates glossary definitions. Illustrations (figures and tables) are comprehensively referred to from the text. Therefore, significant items in illustrations have only been given a page reference in the absence of their concomitant mention in the text referring to that illustration.

release, 166
tapping, 148
side-angle pose, Warrior II and, 159–162
side bend in sukhasana, 135–136
side lying legs 90 degrees, 115
sighing, 21
singing bowls, 80
sitali, 94–95, **207**
sitting
    on floor (asanas), 131–138
    moving towards standing position from, 112–113
    see also chair
skin stretching, 47
sleep, preparing for, 189-192
smiling, 53–54
so ham, 79, 81, **206**
sole raises (seated), 125
sounds
    in brahmari breathing, 91
    joint, 58
    in mantras, 23, 79–81
    muladhara chakra, 24–25
    throat chakra, 27
Sovik, Rol, 22, 81
space, creating the maximum, 178
spinal cord, 62
spinal nerves, 43
spine
    fractures, 56
    lubricating, 131–139, 191
    mobilising, 184
    neutral/natural curves, 61–63
    vertebrae, 43, 56, 61, 98–99, 141
standing, 149–174
    asanas, 149–174
    moving from sitting position towards, 112–113
    noticing how it feels, 59
    see also feet; legs
static postures, 58–59, 60
straps and belts, 69, 70
    breathing practice, 140
    bridge (supported), 179
    dynamic calf strengthening, 152
    dynamic chair, 153
    hamstring release, 129

supta baddha konasana (supported), 178
strengthening
    bone, 42, 55–64
    calf, 152
    5-min.
      standing, 149–167
      supine, 110–119
    muscles *see* muscles
    neck, 110
    visualising, 64
stress, 49–54, 61
    acute, 49, 52
    chronic, 49, 52
    energy and, 20
    immune system and, 49–54
stress hormones, 49, 50
stretching
    figure-of-four stretch, 117–119
    muscles, 57
      hamstrings, 130
    skin, 47
stroke (brain), 15–16, 64
sukhasana, **207**
    side bend, 135–136
supine practices, 101–130
supta baddha konasana, 109–110, **207**
    supported, 178
surgery, 60
sushumna nadi, 12, 19, **207**
sutras, 85, **207**
svadisthana chakra, 25, **207**
Svatmarama, 19
sympathetic nervous system, 39, 50, 51
    digestion and, 44

tadasana (mountain pose), **207**
    block support, 150
tailbone (coccyx), 61, 62
Taittiriya – Upanishad, 10
tapping
    back (lower), 144
    collarbones, 74
    neck, 144, 145
    shoulders, 148
Taylor, Jill Bolte, 15–16

thigh(s)
    crossing, 126, 127
    inner, release, 126, 127
third eye (ajna) chakra, 27–28, **203**
thoracic duct, 46, 178
thoracic spine, 61
throat (vishuddha) chakra, 26, **208**
time (for practice), making, 3–4, 7–8, 65
toes, opening, 131–132
tongue curling or circling, 94–95
transverse abdominal muscles, 38
trauma (traumatic event), 10, 51, 52
    disconnection in, 11, 51
    recovery, 52
tree pose, horse stance to, 163–164
triangle pose (trikonasana), 171–172, 174, **207**
trikonasana, 171–172, 174, **207**
Turner, Kelly A, 16–17
twists/twisting
    balance twist, 170
    dynamic lunge (Warrior II with twists), 157
    framed supine twist, 123–124
    goalpost twists, 138
    safe practice, 56–57
    to stimulate samana vayu, 106–110

udana/udana vayu, 19, 23, 30, **207**, 200
    mudras supporting, 78
union
    immune system and, 41–47
    meaning, 10
    of mind and body, 200
    see also connection
universal mantras, 80–81

vagus nerve, 39–40, 51–52
    dorsal, 51, 52
    mouth/tongue stimulating and, 95
    ventral, 51, 52
vajra mudra, 77, **200**
vam, 25

van der Kolk, Bessel, 52
vayus, **208**
    apana vayu *see* apana vayu
    prana vayu, 19–21, 200
    samana vayu *see* samana vayu
    stimulating, 23–24
    udana vayu *see* udana
    vyana vayu *see* vyana vayu
vertebrae, 43, 56, 61, 98–99, 141
vibrations, 23, 24, 80, 91
    see also humming
vijnyanamaya kosha (intuitive layer of body), 16–17,
    208
viloma, 92–94, **208**
viparita karani, **208**
    with blankets, 175–176
    see also wall support
vishuddha chakra, 26–27, **208**
visualising, building strength, 64
vital energy *see* prana
vyana vayu, 19, 22–23, 30, 36, **208**
    mudras supporting, 77

waking up, 183-188
wall support (legs up wall), 128, 176, 200
    figure-of-four stretch, 117, 119
    see also viparita karani
Warrior I, 155-157
Warrior II, dynamic, 159–162
white blood cells, 42, 45–46, 49, 177
wind-relieving pose *see* apanasana

yam, 26
yoga (basics), 1–8
    asanas, $ asanas
    finding time for, 3–4
    immune system and, 47
    meaning, **208**
    props, 69–71
    restorative practices *see* restorative practices
Yoga Sutras of Patanjali, 85

Note: Bold indicates glossary definitions. Illustrations (figures and tables) are comprehensively referred to from the text. Therefore, significant items in illustrations have only been given a page reference in the absence of their concomitant mention in the text referring to that illustration.

The Bowel Cancer Recovery Toolkit

By Sarah Russell

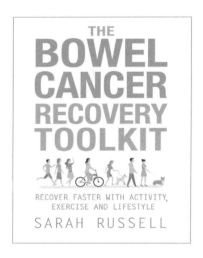

A practical guide to exercising before and after abdominal surgery, especially for cancer, looking at what is safe and effective and what other lifestyle strategies will work with movement and exercise to mitigate the effects of cancer treatment and lower the risk of recurrence.

'Sarah's book is a fantastic starting point for someone living with or beyond colorectal cancer who wants to find out more about exercise during and after cancer treatment. Being active is one of the biggest things you can do to improve your experience and this book will help you achieve that.'

Dr Lucy Gossage, oncologist, triathlete, editor of www.cancerfit.me

Get Your Oomph Back

A guide to exercise after a cancer diagnosis

By Carolyn Garritt

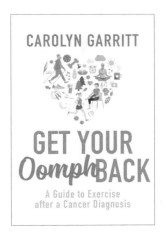

'This is a fantastic book that I wish had been around 13 years ago when I had my own experience of cancer. As a GP I shall be recommending it to patients, and to colleagues who still don't always 'get it' when I talk about the benefits of exercise.'
Dr Jenny Wilson, GP, 5k Your Way Ambassador, cancer survivor

Specialist exercise professional Carolyn Garritt shows how to maximise the benefits of different types of exercise before, during and after treatment for cancer.

Yoga for Cancer
The A to Z of C
By Vicky Fox

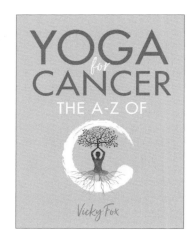

Vicky's wonderful energy, compassion and practical knowledge of supporting people with a cancer diagnosis or history of cancer really shines through in this beautiful book. It is a treasure trove of practical tools and techniques underpinned by a strong philosophy of pain-free working with interoception, truly listening to and supporting the person's needs in the moment.
Dr Nina Fuller-Shavel, Integrative Medicine Doctor, Scientist and Educator

Specialist yoga teacher Vicky Fox's first book shows how to mitigate the side effects of cancer diagnosis and treatment using yoga, starting with A for Anxiety and working through to Z for Zzzz (sleep/insomnia).